NORPLANT: UNDER HER SKIN

NORPLANT: UNDER HER SKIN

Edited by
Barbara Mintzes, Anita Hardon
and Jannemieke Hanhart

Women and Pharmaceuticals Project
WOMEN'S HEALTH ACTION FOUNDATION and WEMOS

Publisher: Eburon
Postbus 2867
2601 CW Delft
The Netherlands

Cover illustration: Thea Boonstra
Cover design: Publish, Amsterdam

In the United States please order directly from:
Boston Women's Health Book Collective
Box 192, West-Somerville, MA 02144, U.S.A.

All other countries please order directly from the publisher or through a bookshop.

The profits from sales of this book will be used to send free copies to organisations in developing countries who are active in the field of women's health. Such copies can be obtained by writing to:

Women's Health Action Foundation
P.O. Box 4263
1009 AG Amsterdam
The Netherlands

CIP-GEGEVENS KONINKLIJKE BIBLIOTHEEK, DEN HAAG

Norplant

Norplant: Under her Skin / ed. by Barbara Mintzes, Anita Hardon and Jannemieke Hanhart. - [S.l]: Women Health Action Foundation; Wemos; [Amsterdam]. Eburon Delft [distr.]
Met lit. opg.
Trefw.: anticonceptiemiddelen.

ISBN 90-5166-299-8

Acknowledgements

We would like to thank Dr. Amal Abd El Hadi, Dr. Aida Seif El Dawla, Judith Richter and others who reviewed drafts of this book. Members of the Women and Pharmaceuticals Project – in particular Janita Janssen, Nicolien Wieringa, Ruth Noyon and Sylvia van Manen – provided extensive advice and direction. Shelley Anderson edited the text and Connie López assisted with administration. We also thank members of the Health Action International (HAI) network and Anthony Arundel for their suggestions and availability for consultation.

We would like to express our thanks to the women who spoke of their experiences with Norplant with the authors of these articles, many of whom were willing to speak openly about intimate sides of their lives and emotionally difficult experiences. We also thank the health workers who described their work and experiences with Norplant, particularly those who did so out of dedication towards better health care for women and better contraceptive services.

Funding for the research and production of this book was provided by Mama Cash, Wilde Ganzen (Wild Geese), the Mission Board of the Dutch Reformed Churches, the Mission and World Service of the Dutch Reformed Churches, Oxfam and the Haella Foundation.

The Directorate General for International Cooperation (DGIS) of the Netherlands Ministry of Foreign Affairs and the European Commission also provided funding for the WEMOS Women and Pharmaceuticals Project while this book was being produced.

WOMEN AND PHARMACEUTICALS PROJECT

The Women and Pharmaceuticals Project was founded in 1985 by WEMOS, a Dutch NGO active in health and development issues, and Health Action International (HAI Europe), an informal network of consumer, health and development groups involved in health and pharmaceutical issues.

WEMOS coordinated the Women and Pharmaceuticals Project from 1985 to 1991. The project aims to enhance the rational use of fertility-related drugs and other drugs used by women through action research, information dissemination and lobbying, in close collaboration with an international network of women's health groups. The Women and Pharmaceuticals Project now works within an independent foundation, the WOMEN'S HEALTH ACTION FOUNDATION.

Table of contents

Introduction

The decision to produce this book was made in the summer of 1989, when women's health activists from Bangladesh, Brazil, India, Indonesia, Thailand, Denmark, Finland and the Netherlands discussed new contraceptive technologies in a meeting sponsored by the Women and Pharmaceuticals Project during the European Women and Health Conference in Madrid.

Norplant, a new contraceptive being heavily promoted for use in family planning programmes, was the main concern of the women who attended this meeting. They wanted to look at Norplant from a user's perspective: does this technology meet the needs of women users? How is it provided to women? Do women's experiences differ in various countries? Are their reproductive rights upheld?

In order to find out more about how women in different societies view the safety and acceptability of Norplant, the Women and Pharmaceuticals Project supported three field studies in Indonesia, Finland and Brazil. These studies were conducted between 1989 and 1991. The results are reported in this book, along with a literature review of studies on users' attitudes to Norplant.

This book does not primarily examine the safety of Norplant from a medical perspective. It examines how women in different societies experience this technology, including their experiences of side-effects which affect sexuality and daily life. Health workers do not always take these side-effects seriously. They tend to reassure women that these are normal effects of the contraceptive and not dangerous, and that they may become less severe with time. However, if women's overall emotional health, social life and sense of well-being are seen as important, then the appraisal of Norplant's appropriateness changes.

What are the characteristics of Norplant?

Norplant is a long-acting hormonal contraceptive consisting of six silicone rods which are implanted under the skin of a woman's upper arm. These rods release levonorgestrel, a synthetic form of the hormone progesterone which is already widely in use in combined oral contraceptives and in the progestin-only mini-pill. Norplant is effective for five years. It requires minor surgery with a local anaesthetic to be inserted or removed, and it must be removed after five years. If it is not removed after five years, the implants continue to release smaller amounts of levonorgestrel. This raises concerns of foetal exposure to levonorgestrel if a woman becomes pregnant or a potentially higher risk of ectopic (tubal) pregnancy, a condition which is life threatening if untreated. If a woman chooses to continue to use the method for longer than five years, she must have a new set of rods inserted.

Many Norplant users experience side-effects. Changes in the pattern of menstrual bleeding are experienced by about 60% of Norplant users in the first year after implantation. This is the most common side-effect caused by Norplant and the most important reason for discontinuing the method (Liskin, et al. 1987).

Distribution of Norplant in family planning programmes

Norplant is mainly used in developing countries. It is currently marketed in 26 countries, most of which are in Asia, Latin America and Africa, and is available within national family planning programmes in two additional countries. About 1.5 million women have used or currently use Norplant[1].

Many of the family planning programmes in which Norplant is distributed have explicit aims to limit population growth. A 1985 World Bank document states that at least 42 countries, comprising more than three quarters of the population of developing countries, have adopted policies to reduce population growth by means of "vigorous family planning programmes" (Ainsworth, 1985).

---

1 **Registration of Norplant 6 x 36 mg levonorgestrel implants**
(Country and year of registration)
Bangladesh (1990), Chile (1988), China (1989), Colombia (1986), Czechoslovakia (1989), Dominican Republic (1985), Ecuador (1985), Finland (1983), Haiti (1989), Indonesia (1985), Jamaica (1992), Kenya (1989), Malaysia (1990), Mali (1992), Mauritius (1991), Mexico (1991), Peru (1987), Rwanda (1992), Singapore (1990), former Soviet Union (1991), Sri Lanka (1987), Sweden (1985), Taiwan (1992), Thailand (1986), USA (1990), Venezuela (1987).
In addition, family planning programmes in two countries (Nepal and Tunisia) have been authorised to provide Norplant. About 1.5 million women have used Norplant in the countries where it has been approved for widespread distribution. Some 55,000 women used Norplant either in clinical or pre-introduction studies (Leiras, 1992; Population Council, 1992).

The emphasis on promotion of contraceptive use in family planning programmes with demographic aims rather than meeting individual women's needs has far-reaching consequences for the services: "Because of the emphasis on getting people to accept a method, follow-up services were minimal and the potential side-effects of the methods were not often explained to clients for fear they would not accept." (Ainsworth, 1985, p. 5).

Because it must be removed surgically, Norplant is prone to abuse if health workers do not respect a woman's wish to have the implants removed or do not provide her with complete information before she has the implants inserted. Several of the articles in this book document both lack of access to full information and difficulties in obtaining removals.

Norplant requires fairly sophisticated health services to be used safely, including sterile technique for insertion and removal, and continued access to health services. Follow-up of Norplant users is more complicated than follow-up of users of most other methods because women need to have the implants removed after five years of use. This type of follow-up is a huge task, especially in areas where the population is not stable due to migration.

How do women in different countries experience Norplant?

The first article in this collection is a literature review of conflicting views on Norplant acceptability based on an analysis of published acceptability studies, and a discussion of the results and limitations in study design from a user's perspective.

The study in Lombok, Indonesia, focuses on how women experience menstrual cycle disturbances caused by Norplant. These experiences are related to cultural ideas about menstruation, an authoritarian social structure and Indonesian family planning policies. The attitudes of family planning workers and the information provided to potential users are discussed.

The Finnish study is important because Finland is the country where Norplant is manufactured and was the first country to approve and market this contraceptive. Norplant's use in Finland gives it credibility in family planning programmes in developing countries. The sample of Finnish health care providers and the experts on Norplant interviewed in this study, however, tend to view Norplant as a contraceptive of second choice. Women tend to ask for the method more often than physicians provide it, often because they have read enthusiastic articles in newspapers and magazines. Counselling is used to give more balanced information and often to dissuade women from using the method.

The article from Brazil presents results of interviews with women who participated in trials of Norplant. Further enrolment in these trials was discontinued in 1986 due to political pressure and concerns about ethical conduct of the trials. A group of 52 women who participated in the trial were interviewed six years later. These women had not been properly followed up after five years of Norplant use and, in some cases, had not been able to find a trained health worker to remove their implants.

Norplant requires specialised training for health workers for proper insertion and removal. The Thai study examines the records of a hospital training session in Thailand. This is a single example in one district hospital. However, the evidence from medical records and an interview points to inadequate record-keeping, lack of follow-up of participants, lack of training in removals and lack of attention to contraindications. The authors question the quality of care received by the women who had Norplant implanted during the training session. They believe that this training session is no exception, and that it illustrates the gap between published Population Council recommendations for how training for Norplant provision should occur and how it may actually be carried out.

The final article highlights the experiences of participants in an introductory trial of Norplant in Egypt and describes the role international donor agencies, scientists and the Egyptian national press play in the promotion of Norplant. Newspaper articles describe Norplant as a "magic capsule" which is both modern and safe. The author's interviews of women participating in the Assiut University trial contrast sharply with these press reports; women speak of side-effects and, in several instances, express anger at family planning physicians' refusal to remove the capsules.

A framework for judging Norplant

The authors of these articles differ in their views of what should be done about Norplant. Some believe that it should be banned because it is a technology which is prone to abuse. Others think that Norplant could be as safe as other commonly used hormonal methods such as the contraceptive pill if it is provided within a good health care service. However, all of the authors have concerns about how Norplant is currently being provided to women, particularly in developing countries.

The figure on the next page provides a framework for viewing contraceptive technologies within a political and socio-cultural context.

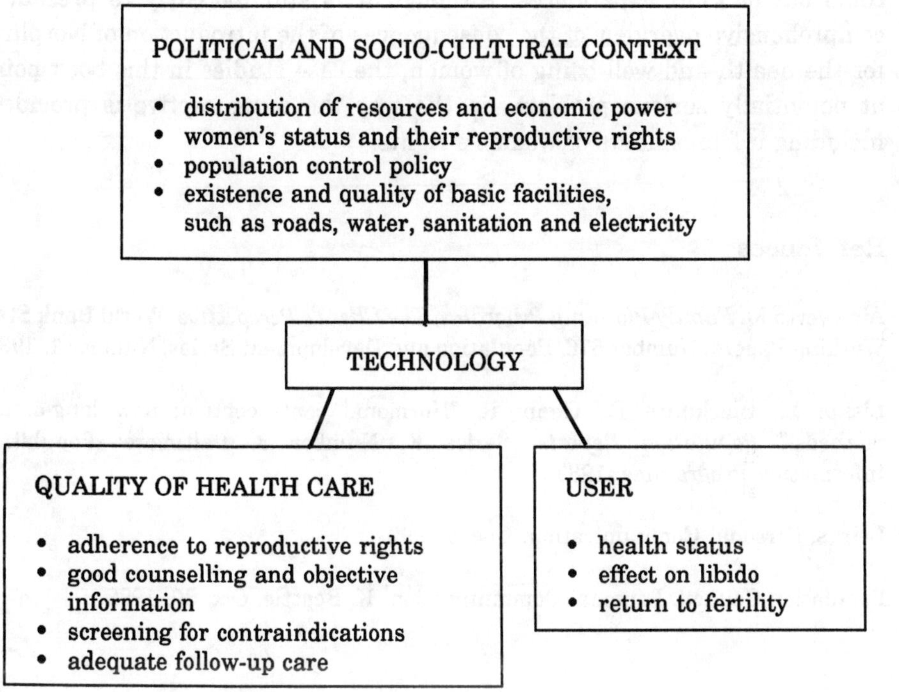

Contraceptives are not simply technical solutions to the prevention of pregnancy; their characteristics affect women's daily lives and social relationships. Technologies whose administration and removal are controlled by a health worker and not the woman herself are inappropriate in settings in which women have a low status and limited rights, and where governments aim to control population growth and therefore women's fertility.

Power relations between North and South, between governments and their people and between men and women all should be considered in evaluating the appropriateness of a technology.

Who was Norplant designed for? Was it for donor aid agencies and family planning programmes who wish to implement a programme as efficiently as possible, and show real results in terms of a lowered birth rate? Was it for the pharmaceutical company which manufactures Norplant and profits from its sales? Or was it for the women who use it and live with its effects daily for up to five years at a time?

If Norplant was designed to meet the needs of the women who use it, then the evaluation of whether Norplant is a "good" contraceptive must ultimately come out of their experiences. Although it is still too early to present a comprehensive overview of the consequences of the introduction of Norplant for the health and well-being of women, the case studies in this book point at potentially serious problems in the way the contraceptive is provided, including infringements of women's rights.

References

Ainsworth M. *Family Planning Programs, The Client's Perspective*. World Bank Staff Working Papers, Number 676. Population and Development Series, Number 1, 1985.

Liskin L., Blackburn R., Ghani R. "Hormonal contraception: new long-acting methods." *Population Reports*, Series K, Number 3. Baltimore: Population Information Programme, 1987.

Leiras. Personal Communication. Dec. 8,1992.

Population Council. Personal Communication. K. Beattie. Oct. 30, 1992.

Norplant: conflicting views on its safety and acceptability

by Anita Hardon

Introduction

The long-acting hormonal contraceptive, Norplant, consists of six silicone-coated rods, each containing 36 mg of the progestin levonorgestrel. When implanted under a woman's skin, the method can prevent pregnancy for five years. It was developed by the Population Council[1] and has been produced by Leiras Pharmaceuticals of Finland since 1983. Norplant has been registered in 26 countries around the world (Population Council 1992; Leiras 1992).

This article reviews the controversies surrounding Norplant's introduction in developing countries. Special attention is given to studies to assess Norplant's acceptability. The design, results, and conclusions of these studies are reviewed with respect to several concerns that have been raised by women's health advocates.

The history of Norplant

Norplant's contraceptive effect was initially based on the principle that a small dose of progestin can suppress fertility without suppressing ovulation. Fewer side-effects, compared to the contraceptive pill, were also expected from implants which could continuously release low doses of progestin. Clinical trials were conducted between 1970 and 1975 to determine the most effective combinations of rods and hormones. The current Norplant system was decided upon in 1974.

1 The Population Council conducts social and health science research relevant to developing countries and biomedical research to develop and improve contraceptive technology.

While testing implants containing megestrol acetate in Chile, Brazil and India, the researchers were confronted with ovarian hypertrophy and an increased number of ectopic pregnancies (pregnancy outside the uterus) among the contraceptive failures. The numbers were higher than would be expected in a comparable group not using contraceptives. These sequelae were caused by the low dose of progestin (Liukko et al. 1977; Segal 1983), which inhibits the transportation of the egg through the fallopian tubes. By 1975 the Population Council decided to increase the dose, thus reducing the chance of pregnancy as well as diminishing the risk of ectopic pregnancy.

The dose of levonorgestrel released by Norplant is approximately 85 micrograms/day in the first few months of use, decreasing gradually to 35 micrograms/day after the first eighteen months and an average of 30 micrograms over the five year period of use (Population Council 1990a). The initial daily dose of levonorgestrel is higher than the daily dose contained in some progestin-only mini-pills such as Microluton, Microval or Norgeston, which contain 30 micrograms of levonorgestrel. The dose of levonorgestrel is lower than that contained in combined oral contraceptives, however.

The first multinational clinical trials[2] of levonorgestrel implants were conducted in 1975 in Brazil, Chile, Denmark, the Dominican Republic, Finland and Jamaica. They were monitored by the International Committee for Contraceptive Research (ICCR), a network of collaborating centres founded by the Population Council. The Population Council chose levonorgestrel as the progestin for their implants because:

> "It was the longest-working reliable progestin, it had already been approved by the FDA and had been used in oral contraceptives since the 1960s, and it had the highest continuation rates (relatively few women had their implant removed within the first three years of use.)" (Segal 1983).

---

2 For an overview of clinical trials on Norplant see references in *Norplant Worldwide. Contraceptive subdermal implants* - a newsletter published by the Population Council.

Mechanisms of action and side-effects[3]

Norplant prevents conception in two ways: by suppressing ovulation in slightly more than 50% of menstrual cycles and by thickening the cervical mucus, so that it is impermeable to sperm. The overall (cumulative) pregnancy rate for the entire five years is only 3.9 per 100 users. This means that during the method's five year period of effectiveness, around four out of every 100 users are likely to become pregnant. The effectiveness of Norplant is correlated with the woman's weight. Heavier women, particularly those who weigh more than 70 kilograms (approximately 154 pounds), have a higher probability of becoming pregnant after the second year of use than lighter women. The cumulative pregnancy rate after five years of use for women weighing over 70 kg is 8.5 per 100 women (WHO 1990).

The contraceptive effect quickly ceases after the implants are removed. According to the Population Council (1990a), pregnancy rates for women who have Norplant removed in order to become pregnant are similar to the rates for women using no contraception.

In a manual for clinicians, the Population Council (1990b) lists the contraindications for Norplant use. These include cardio-vascular disorders, abnormal vaginal bleeding without a known cause, benign or malignant liver tumours, and known or suspected breast cancer. In addition, recently published WHO guidelines warn that women who use Norplant and who have certain conditions such as diabetes, anaemia, or high blood pressure should receive regular medical checkups (WHO 1990).

Both the World Health Organisation (WHO) guidelines and the Population Council manual mention that pregnant women should not use Norplant and that Norplant should not be considered a method of first choice in lactating women. The WHO guidelines recommend that Norplant should not be used until six weeks after giving birth. Both references also advise clinicians to consider whether the woman is a smoker or taking any other medications.

The most frequently reported side-effect, according to both the guidelines and the manual, are changes in menstrual bleeding patterns. Irregularities vary widely and may include, according to a 1990 WHO report: prolonged menstrual bleeding during the first months of use or spotting between periods; no bleeding at all for several months (up to a year or longer in a few cases); or a combination of these patterns.

---

3 *Norplant: A Summary of scientific Data* summarizes the major findings of the clinical trials, pre-introduction studies and some acceptability studies, and contains an extensive bibliography (Population Council 1990a).

In addition, both the manual and guidelines mention other complaints that are likely to be caused by Norplant. These include: dizziness, headache, nervousness, weight gain, ovarian cysts, acne and other skin and hair disorders, and infections at the implant site. The references mention several other complaints that have been reported by users or physicians and which may be associated with Norplant: nipple discharge, inflammation of the cervix, mood changes, depression, general malaise, weight loss, itching and hypertension.

If one or more of the rods break during insertion or removal, as occasionally occurs, women may be accidentally exposed to a higher than recommended dose of progestin.

Concerns about Norplant

Norplant is a complex contraceptive technology which requires a medical professional for administration and removal. Concerns about Norplant were expressed during a meeting of women's health advocates on contraceptive development and use in Woudschoten, the Netherlands, 1991 (Mintzes 1992). A potential for abuse of Norplant exists in family planning programmes that do not acknowledge a woman's right to a choice of birth control methods and her right to have the implants removed whenever she wants. Removal problems have occurred when the rods were not inserted properly, when health personnel were not sufficiently trained in removal or when a fibrous capsule had formed around the rods. There are also concerns about foetal exposure to progestin when the method fails to prevent pregnancy, when the Norplant rods are implanted in pregnant women or when the rods are left in for longer than five years. Furthermore, women's health advocates question the safety of Norplant use by lactating women, particularly directly after childbirth, and they stress the need for more research on the long-term effects of Norplant. In Bangladesh and Brazil, women's health advocates opposed the introduction of Norplant for these reasons. In Brazil, the Ministry of Health stopped further enrolment in an ongoing trial (Gomes dos Reis 1990; Faúndes 1991).

WHO evaluation

In 1985 the World Health Organisation (WHO) presented its evaluation report on Norplant (WHO 1985). The report concluded that Norplant was an "effective and reversible long-term method of fertility regulation...particularly advantageous to women who wish an extended period of contraceptive protection" and that Norplant was "suitable for use in family planning programmes along with other methods of fertility regulation". At the same time, the report pointed out the need for a training programme for medical personnel, more research on long-term side-effects, research into the use of implants during lactation, post-marketing surveillance studies and additional acceptability studies.

In order to learn about rare reactions associated with Norplant use, the WHO, in collaboration with the Population Council and Family Health International, initiated a large-scale surveillance study of Norplant users. The study began in June 1987 with pilot projects in Chile, Sri Lanka and Thailand. The full surveillance project started in the autumn of 1988 at multiple centres in seven countries: Bangladesh, Chile, China, Egypt, Indonesia, Sri Lanka and Thailand. The study follows 7,500 to 8,000 Norplant users and the same number of controls, most of whom use an intrauterine device (IUD), for five years.

Data from all the participating centres in the study are being collected and analyzed at the WHO's headquarters in Geneva. The study also investigates what happens to women if they switch to another method of birth control or become pregnant, and gathers data not only on commonly recorded reactions, but also on rare events such as tubal pregnancies. This type of post-marketing surveillance could not have been conducted before Norplant was in widespread use, because rare and long-term side-effects cannot be detected without a large group of users.

For a few of the effects being studied, it is unfortunate that this large study only compares Norplant users to IUD users. IUD users have a higher frequency of heavy or prolonged menstrual bleeding, intermenstrual bleeding and spotting, and menstrual pain than non-users. If a woman becomes pregnant during IUD use, she has a ten times increased risk that it is an ectopic pregnancy (Guillebaud 1991). Women using IUDs also have a higher risk of developing pelvic inflammatory disease (PID) than non-users. PID in turn leads to higher rates of ectopic pregnancy and infertility (Farley et al., 1992). Because of these IUD-associated risks and the comparison of Norplant users to IUD users, this study is unlikely to show whether Norplant leads to higher rates of ectopic pregnancy, infertility or other health problems caused by menstrual disturbances.

After several studies on lactation, the Population Council now recommends that contraceptives based on steroids, such as Norplant, should not be the first choice for breast-feeding women. Levonorgestrel is present in the milk of women using Norplant while breast-feeding. Studies have shown no significant effects on the growth or health of breast-fed infants whose mothers used levonorgestrel implants beginning six weeks after childbirth, but there is no similar data on the use of Norplant during the six weeks just after birth (Population Council 1990a). These studies have not assessed the long-term effects of exposure to progestins in infancy, which remains unknown. There are reports that Norplant is frequently provided to breast-feeding mothers in developing countries in spite of the Population Council's recommendation against this.

In line with WHO's recommendations, the Population Council initiated research on user-satisfaction with Norplant and the service delivery system through which it is offered. The Population Council reports that user and programme studies are under way in Bangladesh, Brazil, Colombia, the Dominican Republic, Egypt, Ghana, Haiti, Kenya, Indonesia, Mexico, Nepal, Nigeria, the Philippines, Senegal, Singapore, Thailand, the United States and Zambia.

Norplant acceptability studies

More acceptability studies have been conducted on Norplant than on any other contraceptive or fertility regulating method currently available. Tables 1 and 2 give an overview of the aims, methods, results and conclusions of Norplant acceptability studies that have been published during the past decade in two scientific journals: *Studies in Family Planning* and *International Family Planning Perspectives* (Shabaan et al. 1983; Satayapan et al. 1983; Marangoni et al. 1983; Lubis et al. 1983; Basnayake et al. 1988; Darney et al. 1988; Kane et al. 1990; Zimmerman et al. 1990). Studies which have not been published in these two journals are not reviewed here.[4]

Table 1 shows that there is some variation in the stated aims of each study, although all address how users view Norplant. Sometimes additional aims are given, such as studying safety and efficacy, or studying factors that influence acceptability. The number of respondents in each study varies from 205 in a study in San Francisco (Darney 1988) to 2,586 in a four-country study (Kane et al. 1990).

4 This is a limitation of this review, as several other studies have been conducted by the Population Council on service delivery systems and quality of care. The results of these studies have not yet been published and are not publicly available.

Most studies have focused on the acceptability of Norplant to users and to women who discontinued use. One four-country study (Kane et al. 1990) also assessed acceptability to potential users (for example, people coming to a family planning service in search of a suitable contraceptive); and another comparative study (Zimmerman et al. 1990) examined the acceptability of Norplant to husbands and family planning programme personnel.

In all studies except in the study by Zimmerman et al. (1990), the respondents are interviewed in university-based health clinics or mother and child clinics in urban centres, where the service delivery system is likely to be better than in small village clinics. The clinic environment may also have influenced the responses of women to the interview questions. Women are likely to identify the interviewers as health service personnel, and consequently may avoid talking about problems encountered with the service delivery system. An alternative environment for discussing the advantages and disadvantages of specific contraceptives would be the community or the homes of users and non-users. More insights into socio-cultural aspects that affect contraceptive use can be gained in these settings by also interviewing other people involved, such as the user's husband or mother.

N.B.

None of the studies reviewed explicitly stated which criteria and indicators were used to determine the acceptability of a contraceptive. Two implicit criteria appear to have been used: the frequency with which women continued to use the method and the frequency with which women decided to stop using the method because of side-effects (see Table 2).

Details on the inclusion and exclusion criteria used to select the respondents are given in only three studies: in Indonesia (Lubis et al. 1983), Thailand (Satayapan et al. 1983), and Sri Lanka (Basnayake et al. 1988). The other studies do not give details other than that the respondents were 'Norplant users' or 'potential users'. One of the four-country studies (Zimmerman et al. 1990) cautions that, in addition to the formal criteria, other selection processes may occur. The authors report that clinic staff may select women who are likely to keep the implants for the entire five-year period. The pre-introductory trial in Ecuador also reports that clinic staff play a role in client selection:

N.B.

> "Staff were worried mainly about the women's reactions to the pronounced bleeding disturbance associated with the implants.... The staff was initially overselective in choosing users, but as the trial progressed they became more confident and the rate of acceptance increased." (Marangoni et al. 1983, p. 179).

Table 1 Norplant acceptability studies: aims and methods

Country	Aims	Number of respondents	Type of respondents	Research site	Criteria for in/exclusion
Indonesia Lubis et al. 1983	•assess performance of Norplant •provide data on acceptability	813	users	2 urban clinics	PC[a] criteria
Thailand Sataypan et al. 1983	•determine how Norplant is perceived •measure continuation rate	887	users	3 urban clinics	PC criteria
Egypt Shaaban et al. 1983	•evaluate acceptability of Norplant •compare with IUD	250	users	1 urban clinic	not given
Ecuador Marangoni et al. 1983	•determine acceptability of Norplant	283	users	2 urban clinics	not given
Sri Lanka Basnayake et al. 1988	•evaluate safety, efficacy, and acceptability of Norplant	400	users	2 urban clinics	married 18-40 years no contraindications not pregnant
USA Darney et al. 1988	•identify personal perceptions of Norplant •define determinants of and levels of user-satisfaction	205	users	1 urban clinic	not given
Four country I Kane et al. 1990	•determine level of interest in trying Norplant •determine impact of social and demographic factors	2586	potential users	10 clinics	start/change contraceptive use
Four country II Zimmerman et al. 1990	•look at Norplant from perspective of users and nonusers •understanding concerns and motivations of users	279	users nonusers husbands service providers in focus group discussions	urban clinics	countries with more than five years experience with Norplant no specifics on selection of participants in focus group discussions

[a] Population Council

Table 2 Norplant acceptability studies: main results and conclusions

Country	1-year continuation rate	Main reasons for discontinuing	Main side-effects	% of users	Other important results	Conclusion
Indonesia Lubis et al. 1983	95.3	•menstrual problem •skin problem •husband objection	irregular menstruation amenorrhoea skin irritation	52 21 11	frequency of side-effects increases with education	Norplant may be acceptable to women
Thailand Satayapan et al. 1983	88.4	•menstrual problem •skin infection •other medical reasons	menstrual change headache depression	57 6 2	11% of discontinuation is due to infections at implant site	Results are strong indication of acceptability
Egypt Shaaban et al. 1983	89.6	•bleeding/pain •personal •pregnancy	menstrual change headache depression	67[a] 6 1	continuation rate - Norplant is better than IUD	Norplant is an acceptable method that deserves wider use.
Ecuador Marangoni et al. 1983	87.4	•menstrual problem •skin infection •acne and headache	not given		first few removals proved to be difficult	There is substantial demand for a contraceptive like Norplant
Sri Lanka Basnayake et al. 1988	98.7	•pregnancy •menstrual problem	menstrual change headache and dizziness back, stomach pain	71.8[b] 19 16	40% users mention long-acting effect as advantage of Norplant	The study suggests that Norplant is a safe, effective, acceptable method
USA Darney et al. 1988	2-year rate 77	•side-effects •fears inefficacy (end of 5 years) •medical reasons	menstrual change weight change headache	82 32 24	other side-effects include decreased libido, chest pains, numbness of arms	This study found Norplant an acceptable method of contraception
Four country I Kane et al. 1990	no data	*reasons not to try Norplant*: prefer other method fear of side-effects husband disapproves			*reported advantages of Norplant*: effectiveness newness promise safety	The study reveals a relatively high level of interest in using Norplant
Four country II Zimmerman et al. 1990	no data	*perceived disadvantages*: irregular, prolonged bleeding weight loss headache dizziness			*rumours in all countries*: causes sterility and cancer capsules migrate affects breast milk reports that removal on demand does not always occur to satisfaction of user	Findings permit programme planners to identify resistance points

[a] At 3-month follow-up. At 12-month follow-up this was 30%.
[b] This was at 3-month follow-up. At 12 months 75% complained of menstrual change.

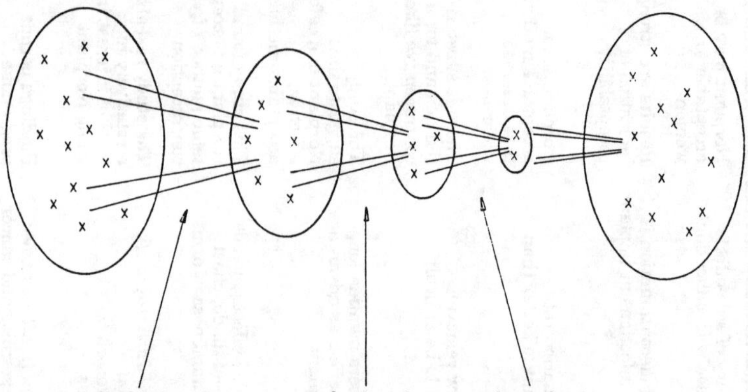

Figure 1 The selection of a research population in acceptability studies

Figure 1 summarizes the selection process for users and non-users in the Norplant acceptability studies. The figure shows that the study population is far from representative of the general population that will use the method once it is marketed and distributed through health care channels. Despite this methodological shortcoming, the authors of these studies tend to draw conclusions, such as the following, about the acceptability of Norplant to users (see also Table 2):

> "The data presented in this article are encouraging and indicate that Norplant implants may be acceptable to Indonesian women." (Lubis et al. 1983, p. 183).

> "We interpret these continuation rates, and the perceptions and experiences of the users of the method to date, as a strong indication of the acceptability of the implant methods." (Satayapan et al. 1983, p. 176).

> "Norplant implants are an effective acceptable method of contraception with minimal side-effects, and definitely deserve wider use in Egypt." (Shaaban et al. 1983, p. 167).

> "Our experience shows that there is a substantial demand for a contraceptive with the characteristics of the Norplant system..." (Marangoni et al. 1983, p. 179).

> "The study of 205 women who received Norplant contraceptives at an urban family planning clinic in the USA found Norplant to be a highly acceptable method of contraception for women of different ethnic and economic groups, despite the occurrence of side-effects." (Darney et al. 1990, p. 158).

In addition to the problem of how closely the study participants represent most potential users, the absence of explicit indicators and criteria for determining acceptability makes it difficult to judge the validity of the general conclusion that Norplant is an acceptable contraceptive for a wider population.

The acceptability studies report relatively high continuation rates. Menstrual changes, skin irritation and headaches are reported to be the main side-effects and the main reasons for discontinuing Norplant use. In interpreting the results, the authors tend to define disorders such as headaches, dizziness and weight gain as minor problems with no proven link to Norplant. The Sri Lankan acceptability study, for example, reports:

> "Of the 189 women who were followed up at 12 months, one reported that she had been hospitalised for prolonged headache and dizziness, [but] no medical problems could be found." (Basnayake et al. 1988, p. 43).

Women's fears of long-term health effects or effects on the foetus are classified as rumours that act as obstacles to the expansion of Norplant use. One study states that the "rumours reported by participants in all countries" were that:

> "1) Norplant causes cancer and sterility, 2) the capsules migrate to other parts of the body, and 3) the breast milk of Norplant users negatively affects offspring." (Zimmerman et al. 1990, p. 97).

Understanding the user's perspective

Perhaps the most important limitation of the Norplant acceptability studies is their failure to investigate the participants' beliefs concerning reproductive physiology, their perception of the mode of action of the various contraceptive methods, and their evaluation of a birth control method's costs and benefits. Beliefs about reproductive physiology clearly affect people's perceptions of each contraceptive method. For example, Nichter et al. (1989), in an essay on modern fertility regulating methods, explains how many Sri Lankans explain the effects of oral contraceptives:

> "A pervasive notion among informants was that the pill worked because of its heating effect in the body....Some informants noted that taking these pills every day raised the heat level of the body to such an extent that male and female *dhatu*, a substance associated with vitality and strength, was burned up....Another health concern noted by Sinhalese women was that the excess heat in a woman's body caused by taking the pill rendered the womb dry. Over time a dry womb becomes incapable of accepting male seed."

Nichter stresses that the issues of "rumours" and "side-effects" need to be addressed by a more profound analysis of why these concerns exist.

It is remarkable that so little has been written about the consequences of menstrual disturbances on the day-to-day life of Norplant users. Anthropological research suggests that the consequences can be far-reaching. Menstruation is an important event in any woman's life. The presence or absence of menstruation affects a wide range of activities such as cooking procedures, sexual interactions and religious practices (Buckley et al. 1988; WHO 1981; DelVecchio Good 1977). Douglas has described how menstrual blood is often perceived to be a dangerous element for men (1988, p. 147). Among the Enga of New Guinea, for example:

> "Contact with it, or with a menstruating woman will, in the absence of appropriate counter-magic, sicken a man and cause persistent vomiting, "kill" his blood so that it turns black, corrupt his vital juices so that his skin darkens and hangs in folds as his flesh wastes, permanently dull his wits, and eventually lead to a slow decline and death."

Many societies consider the delay or absence of menstruation to be unhealthy for a woman (Newman 1985). In Columbia, Browner (1985) found that lack of menstruation is perceived as an illness. Ngin (1985) reported that many Chinese Malays believe that irregular menstruation is unclean and bad for a woman's health and that remedies should be taken to ensure the expected onset of bleeding. Laderman (1983) notes that women in East Malaysia are encouraged to eat sweet foods to increase the flow of scanty menstruation. In addition, menstruating women in East Malaysia cannot pray during menses and men are not supposed to have sexual intercourse with their wives at this time.

The developers of Norplant have a technical answer to the irregular menstruation resulting from Norplant use. They recommend that potential users be counselled about the possibility of suffering from menstrual disorders, especially in the first few months after Norplant implantation, and that they be told that this adverse effect is not medically serious and that haemoglobin levels do not decrease (WHO 1990; Population Council 1990b).

How the technology affects the user-provider relationship

Another limitation of the acceptability studies is that they do not examine how the new Norplant technology affects the relationship between the provider and the user. Women are dependent on health workers for removal of Norplant, and thus for the reversal of its effects. There are reports of providers refusing to remove the implants despite requests from women participating in the pre-introductory trials. The 1990 report on the four-country accessibility study discussed this problem:

> "In all four countries there were reports that removal on demand did not occur to the satisfaction of the user. Women participating in the clinical study who asked for removal because of irregular bleeding experienced the greatest difficulty, as clinicians often suggested waiting to see whether the menstrual flow would normalize. Both service providers and discontinuers reported that when faced with a clinician that would not remove the implants, women in the Dominican Republic, Egypt and Indonesia learned to give reasons that they knew the clinician would accept, such as the spouse's requesting another baby. In Thailand, because of the cost of the method, women are routinely informed when choosing Norplant that the implants are appropriate for long-term spacing and will not be removed for minor side-effects." (Zimmerman et al. 1990, p. 99).

These findings are alarming, particularly in a study which recommends the introduction of Norplant. They can be understood in part by considering the different interests of the providers and users. There are several reasons why family planning workers and clinicians could be interested in achieving high continuation rates. For example, the cost of Norplant has been used in Thailand as a reason to discourage removal upon request. Another reason is the preoccupation of family planning programmes with achieving low fertility rates. Clinicians who personally identify with the trials' success may promote "high continuation rates" as a sign of a successful outcome.

Information provision and contraceptive choice

None of the acceptability studies describe the information that was provided to women about Norplant prior to acceptance of the method, even though this information is likely to affect a woman's perception of the method's effects and side-effects. The Ecuadorian study does refer to this information, but gives no details about its content:

> "The professionally designed educational materials directed to both the users and the clinic personnel were especially effective informational tools." (Marangoni et al. 1983, p. 179).

Since information on the content of the "effective informational tools" is not provided, it is impossible to determine if women were adequately informed about other birth control methods and their relative advantages and disadvantages. Nor is it clear if the trials followed appropriate procedures for informed consent.

One recently published study on information provision should be mentioned here. This is a study by Hardy and Goodson (1992) that compared Norplant and IUD acceptors (with no contraindications for Norplant use) on their perception of the information received at the family planning clinic. The two groups had received exactly the same information on both methods in a group counselling session. The IUD acceptors group, however, recalled much less information on Norplant than the Norplant acceptors group. The researchers stress that one important factor in explaining this difference is the method preference of the respondents prior to coming to the clinic. Eighty-two percent of the Norplant acceptors had heard about the method before coming to the clinic. Information sources other than the family planning clinics probably helped to determine which method each woman chose.

Health groups and women in Bangladesh and Brazil have seriously criticized the acceptability studies of Norplant (UBINIG 1988; Gomes dos Reis 1990). One criticism is that these trials do not genuinely test the acceptability of the method. Instead, they appear to be designed to overcome resistance to Norplant and to provide advance marketing. A 1981 newspaper article in Bangladesh, calling for participants to take part in a trial of Norplant, described Norplant as "A new birth control method, ... A wonderful innovation of modern science [that] can be implanted under the skin of the arm, [it] will ensure sterility for five years [and] when removed, [one] can have children again." (UBINIG 1988).

The potential for abuse

Women cannot remove Norplant themselves; they are dependent on a health worker. If the health worker refuses or if they are not given an informed choice of birth control methods before having Norplant inserted, they lose control over an important aspect of their reproductive life. Women's health advocates from many countries are extremely concerned about the potential for abuse which is built into Norplant's design.

These concerns are not unrealistic, as shown by a number of widely publicized cases in the United States that occurred shortly after Norplant's approval by the US Food and Drug Administration in December 1990. The first, and perhaps most serious case, is a Kansas state legislator's proposal to pay US $500 to any welfare mother who uses Norplant. Under the bill, believed to be the first of its kind, the state of Kansas would also pay for implanting the device and for annual checkups. The rationale for the bill, according to sponsor Kerry Leawood, is to save tax payers' money. An estimated US $ 205,000 in public assistance money is spent to support each child in a family on welfare, from birth to adulthood. Leawood stated that "something has to be done to reduce the number of unwanted pregnancies, and this type of voluntary programme, where the public is given a strong financial incentive to use a safe reversible contraceptive device that has a useful life of five years represents the best way to prevent them" (Lewin 1991). While this bill had little chance of passing, it demonstrates the potential for the abuse of Norplant. Clearly, providing certain population groups such as welfare mothers with incentives to use specified contraceptive methods interferes with the legal right of all Americans to decide whether or not to practice birth control. The legislation proposed by Leawood could be considered a sanction against welfare mothers who do not wish to use the method.

Another controversial US case was Judge Howard Broadman's order for a woman to have Norplant implanted as part of a plea bargain after she had pleaded guilty to child abuse. The woman was ordered to have the rods inserted after her release from jail and to keep the implants for the entire probation period. In sentencing the woman, the judge made Norplant sound as simple as a condom. "It's a new thing", he said, and "easily removable" (Cantwell 1991).

Upon hearing this, one of the original developers of Norplant, Dr. Sheldon Segal, protested against the infringement of the defendant's reproductive rights (*CDRR News* 1991). Other critics protested that the defendant could have sound medical reasons that would make her use of Norplant harmful. The judge responded by leaving it up to the doctors to decide whether the device would be safe or not (MacKenzie 1991).

In both cases, incentives for women to use Norplant, either money or a shorter jail sentence, were proposed. These incentives interfere with a woman's reproductive rights. In the second case, the fact that doctors were given the right to decide if the method was suitable for the woman confirms women's health advocates' fears about the provider-dependent nature of the method. The woman's own views on a suitable contraceptive were not considered.

It is disturbing that these problems arose so quickly after Norplant's approval in the United States. Other abuses of Norplant could occur in poverty stricken countries where family planning programmes have an explicit mandate to reduce population growth, not for the benefit of the individual, but in the name of state development. Though not yet systematically documented, the introduction of Norplant in these countries is likely to negatively affect the right of women, and men, to free and informed choices about birth control methods.

Conclusion

Women's health advocates are justifiably concerned about the widespread distribution of Norplant to family planning programmes in developing countries before problems concerning its ethical administration, safety, and the provision of adequate service delivery have been resolved. In particular, the appropriate use of a new contraceptive technology such as Norplant depends on the context in which the method is used. A woman's right to freely choose from a range of contraceptives and her right to stop using a contraceptive are likely to be violated if Norplant is administered in a coercive family planning programme.

Norplant is a sophisticated technology that, if it is to be administered safely, requires a high standard of health care. It is questionable whether such standards can be achieved in developing countries. In addition, many women in developing countries who live in remote areas are more likely to suffer from anaemia and to have, or have had, liver diseases. These conditions, which require extra medical attention, make the rational use of Norplant implants especially difficult.

Before distributing Norplant on a wider scale, the long-term health, economic, and social consequences of its use need to be examined and the prerequisites and conditions for safe use determined. This has not been done in the acceptability studies that have been published to date.[5]

The WHO's large surveillance study will produce substantial information on the health-related consequences of Norplant use. However, due to the study's design some questions will remain unanswered. The economic and social consequences of Norplant's introduction do not appear to have been studied as rigorously. One wonders, for example, how the extensive training required for the safe delivery and use of Norplant will be financed. Can training be sustained when the initial international funding stops? Will the financial costs of Norplant for family planning programmes in developing countries lead to a deterioration of other services? These issues have also been raised in the United States. In a review of Norplant, the *Contraceptive Technology Update* (1991) comments that "perhaps the most significant is the problem of cost." The review points out that Norplant's price, approximately US $ 300 for the device, plus insertion and removal costs, will prevent many low-income women from using it.

Safe use appears to be dependent upon the continuous monitoring of Norplant users, following the guidelines of the Population Council and the WHO. The economic consequences of monitoring and supervision also need to be assessed. Two social issues require additional attention: the ethical issue of a woman's right to removal of the implants, particularly in relatively aggressive family planning programmes; and a women's right to objective and balanced information on all contraceptive options. The social and cultural consequences of menstrual disturbances also require systematic attention. Finally, women's health advocates and users from a variety of socio-cultural settings should be involved early on in determining the conditions and prerequisites for Norplant's safe use.

References

Anonymous "Arrival of Norplant may be bittersweet for clinics." *Contraceptive Technology Update* 1991; 12:1-5.

Anonymous "Norplant Easy to Use, Easier to Abuse." *CDRR News*, Jan/Feb. 1991.

---

5 The still-to-be-published studies on service delivery system and quality of care of the Population Council are likely to include information on these aspects of Norplant use and distribution.

Basnayake S., Thalpa S., Balogh S.A. "Evaluation of Safety, Efficacy and Acceptability of Norplant Implants in Sri Lanka." *Studies in Family Planning* 1988; 19:39-47.

Beattie K. "Introduction of New Contraceptive Methods: An Opportunity for Promoting the User's Perspective in Family Planning Programmes." *A Question of Control.* Ed. Barbara Mintzes. WEMOS/HAI, 1992.

Browner C.H. "Traditional Techniques for Diagnosis, Treatment and Control of Pregnancy in Cali, Columbia." In: *Women's Medicine: a Cross-cultural Study of Indigenous Fertility Regulation.* Ed. L.F. Newman. New Brunswick, New Jersey: Rutgers University Press, 1985: 99-124.

Buckley T., Gottlieb A.A. (eds.) *Blood Magic: the Anthropology of Menstruation.* Berkeley: University of California Press, 1988.

Cantwell M., "Coercion and contraception." *New York Times*, 27 January 1991; E16.

Darney P.D., Atkinson E., Tanner S., et al. "Acceptance and perceptions of Norplant among users in San Francisco, USA." *Studies in Family Planning* 1988; 21:153-160.

DelVecchio Good M., "Of Blood and Babies: the Relationship of Popular Islamic Physiology to Fertility." *Social Science and Medicine* 1977; 14B:147-156.

Douglas M., *Purity and Danger: an Analysis of Concepts of Pollution and Taboo.* London: Ark Paperbacks, 1988.

Farley T.M.M., Rosenberg M.J., et al. "Intrauterine Devices and Pelvic Inflammatory Disease: An International Perspective." *Lancet* 28 Mar 1992; 339 (8796): 785-788.

Faúndes A., 1991. "Correspondence on Norplant". *Issues in Reproductive and Genetic Engineering* 1992; 5(1): 67-70.

Gomes dos Reis A.R. "Norplant in Brazil: Implantation Strategy in the Guise of Scientific Research." *Issues in Reproductive and Genetic Engineering* 1990; 3(2):111-119.

Guillebaud J. *Contraception: Your Questions Answered.* Revised ed. London: Churchill Livingstone, 1991.

Hansen E.B., Launso L. "Development, use and evaluation of drugs: the dominating technology." [Figure 1 in this publication is based on Figure 2 in Hansen and Launso] *Social Science and Medicine* 1987; 25:65-73.

Hardy E., Goodson P. "Association between contraceptive method and perception of information received: a comparison of Norplant and IUD acceptors." *Contraception* 43(2): 131-137.

Kane T.T., Farr G., Janowitz B. "Initial acceptability of contraceptive implants in four developing countries." *International Family Planning Perspective* 1990; 16:49-54.

Laderman C. *Childbirth and Nutrition in Rural Malaysia*. Berkeley: University of California Press, 1983.

Leiras. Personal Communication. Dec. 8, 1992.

Lewin T. "A Plan to Pay Welfare Mothers for Birth Control." *New York Times*, 11 Feb. 1991.

Liukko P., et al. "Ectopic pregnancy during use of low-dose progestagens for oral contraception." *Contraception* 1977; 16:575-580.

Lubis F.J., Prihartono T., Agoestina, et al. "One-year experience with Norplant implants in Indonesia. *Studies in Family Planning* 1983; 14:181-184.

Marangoni P., Cartagena S., Alvarado J., et al. "Norplant implants and the TCu 200 IUD: A comparative study in Ecuador." *Studies in Family Planning* 1983; 14:177-180.

MacKenzie J.P. "Whose Choice is It Anyway?" *New York Times*, 1 Jan. 1991.

Newman L.F. *Women's Medicine: a Cross-cultural Study of Indigenous Fertility Regulation*. New Brunswick, New Jersey: Rutgers University Press, 1985.

Ngin C. "Indigenous fertility regulating methods among two Chinese communities in Malaysia." In: *Women's Medicine: a Cross-cultural Study of Indigenous Fertility Regulation*. Ed. L.F. Newman. New Brunswick, New Jersey: Rutgers University Press 1985: 25-42.

Nichter M., Nichter M., "Modern methods of fertility regulation: when and for whom are they appropriate?" In: *Anthropology and International Health*. Ed. M. Nichter. South Asian Case Studies, Dordrecht: Kluwer; 1989: 30-57.

Population Council. "Approvals rise to 15 countries." *Norplant Worldwide*, 14 May 1990. New York: The Population Council.

Population Council. *Norplant. A summary of Scientific Data*. New York: The Population Council, 1990a.

Population Council. *Norplant Contraceptive Subdermal Implant: Manual for Clinicians*. New York: The Population Council, 1990b.

Population Council. *Personal Communication*. K. Beattie. October 30, 1992.

Satayapan S., Kanchanasinith K., Varakamin S. "Perceptions and acceptability of Norplant implants in Thailand." *Studies in Family Planning* 1983; 14:170-176.

Segal S.J. "The development of Norplant implants." *Studies in Family Planning* 1983; 14:159-163.

Shaaban S.M.M., Salah M., Zarzour A., et al. "A prospective study of Norplant implants and the TCu 380Ag IUD in Assiut, Egypt." *Studies in Family Planning* 1983; 14:163-169.

UBINIG. "The Norplant trial: an investigative study on the methodology and ethical issues." *Hygiea* 1988; 3:19-34.

WHO (World Health Organisation) Task Force on Psychosocial Research in Family Planning. "A Cross-cultural Study of Menstruation: Implications for Contraceptive Development and Use." *Studies in Family Planning* 1981; 12:3-16.

WHO (World Health Organisation). "Facts about an implantable contraceptive." *WHO Bulletin* 1985; 33:485-494.

WHO (World Health Organisation). *Norplant Contraceptive Subdermal Implants. Managerial and Technical Guidelines*. Geneva: World Health Organisation, 1990.

Zimmerman M., Haffey J., Crane E., Szumowsky D., Alvarez F., Bhiromrut P., Brache V., Lubis F., Salah M., Shaaban M., Shawky B., Poernomo Sigit Sidi J., "Assessing the acceptability of Norplant implants in four countries: findings from focus group discussions." *Studies in Family Planning* 1990; 21:93-103.

Acknowledgements

Parts of the data presented in this article have been included in papers submitted for publication to the *Anthology on Reproductive Technology* (edited by Helen Bequart Holmes) and to *Social Science and Medicine*. Sandra Waldman of the Population Council, Joanne Spicehandler of the Human Reproduction Programme of the WHO and Judy Norsigan of the Boston Women's Health Book Collective have contributed significantly to this article by sending detailed information and a commentary on earlier drafts.

Women's views on Norplant: a study from Lombok, Indonesia[1]

by Jannemieke Hanhart

Norplant's introduction into Indonesia's Family Planning Programme

The Indonesian government started a family planning programme in 1968. In general the programme is considered to be a success and is used as an example for other countries. Its success stems from the way the campaign has been set up: existing social structures and organisations are used and the target group is often approached in a personal way by means of house-to-house visits. The campaign is also supported by the mass media, political parties and religious organisations. Targets are set by the National Family Planning Board (Badan Koordinasi Keluarga Berencana Nasional – BKKBN), a central government organisation with overall responsibility for family planning. Annual BKKBN plans are linked to the Indonesian Five Year Plans and have established quantified targets for achievement of contraceptive prevalence.

All provinces have a corresponding BKKBN organisation. The provinces have units at the regency, district and subdistrict levels, all of which are responsible through the hierarchy to the central level in Jakarta (Ward et al. 1990, p. 4). The responsibility to reach targets is shared by all community leaders to the lowest level via a top-down model. A combination of individual persuasion and community pressure is used to bring the population to participate in the family planning programme (Warwick 1986).

Norplant was first introduced into Indonesia in 1981 and has since been the subject of several introductory studies (Affandi 1987; Affandi et al. 1987; Lubis 1983; Sutedi n.d.). On the basis of these studies, Norplant was registered in Indonesia in 1986 and accepted into the national family

1 I would like to thank Dr. Firman Lubis, Dr. Ieda Poernomo Sigit Sidi of Yayasan Kusuma Buana, Dr. L. M. Saleh and family and R. Gedarip and family. I am greatly indebted to them for their continuous help and support throughout this fieldwork.

planning programme in 1987. The aim is to use it in all family planning service centres which meet certain requirements.

As a delicate and long-lasting contraceptive, Norplant requires additional training for health workers, including training in insertions, removal, information provision and communication. Additionally, special handling for supply and distribution is required. Instruments for insertions and removals must be available in sufficient numbers and sterile technique must be used (Poernomo Sigit Sidi 1989). The centre must also be able to manage the administrative side of provision and follow-up of users. In Bayan, the region in which this study took place, health centres at a subdistrict level but not at the village level were able to provide Norplant.

Long-lasting contraceptives like Norplant, the IUD and sterilisation are given priority within the family planning programme. The Indonesian family planning programme is the largest provider of Norplant in the world with 350,000 users in 1988 and current estimates of approximately 800,000 users.

This is the target population for Norplant as defined by the policy guidelines of the Indonesian family planning programme:

1. mothers between 20 and 25 years of age, to space their births after weaning;
2. mothers above 30 years of age, to block their fecundity or prevent further births. In this case the use of Norplant becomes a means of durable, but reversible contraception, as an alternative to sterilisation.

Previous studies of experiences with Norplant in Indonesia

Yayasan Kusuma Buana (YKB), a private Indonesian health and family planning foundation, has conducted several studies on the introduction and implementation of Norplant in Indonesia (Poernomo Sigit Sidi 1990; Prihartono 1990; Ward et al. 1990; YKB 1986, 1988; Zimmerman et al. 1990). To improve the quality of services the YKB has developed information and educational materials to train Norplant providers and information materials to inform prospective users of Norplant or other methods of contraception.

In 1986 the YKB carried out a Norplant acceptability study which was part of a four country acceptability study commissioned by the Population Council. The results have been published together with results from Egypt, the Dominican Republic and Thailand by Zimmerman et al. (1990). The studies are qualitative in design and attempt to assess experiences with Norplant, knowledge of the method and attitudes towards it.

Another important study, also commissioned by the Population Council, focuses on service delivery and how Norplant has been implemented in Indonesia. It deals with questions like quality of care, freedom of choice and removal on demand (Ward et al. 1990).

In most studies bleeding problems are mentioned as the most common side-effect and an important reason for dissatisfaction. However, these bleeding problems are not studied in any detail, and the user's view is absent. The acceptability study by Zimmerman et al. (1990) is one of the first to address the user's perceptions and experiences with the implant. Bleeding problems are mentioned and dealt with in some detail, but their effect on the user's life is still not studied in depth.

This study's goals: an in-depth look at the user's experience

This study looks at the user's perspective on bleeding problems in greater depth. These questions form the focus of the study:

- How do women deal with changes in their menstrual cycle caused by contraceptives?
- How do women who use Norplant perceive changes in their menstrual cycle?
- What do these changes mean physically and psychologically?
- How do they affect women's social lives and their sexual relationships?
- What kind of treatment or help do women seek (clinical, traditional, self-medication)? What kind of treatment do they receive?

A second focus is the communication between prospective and current Norplant users and health and family planning workers.

Research area

The fieldwork was conducted from Septemer 1990 until February 1991 in the subdistrict of Bayan located in the northern part of Lombok. It is an agricultural region with some fertile areas, but also with large very dry areas. Farming is mixed and is partially oriented towards subsistence. Most farmers own animals, including buffaloes, cows and goats, and land which they work themselves. The main crops are rice, peanuts, onions, some garlic, maize, coconuts, mangos and rose-apples (*jambu*).

Bayan is the centre of the Wetu Telu, the original Sasak people. Their religion is basically Islam, but is influenced by Hindu and animistic traditions. The *adat*, a set of traditional customs and beliefs, is still very strong. The level of education is low. The main diseases are malaria, diarrhoea, respiratory illnesses and *panas* (fever) which can be partially attributed to malaria. Infant mortality is high. Although the people are beginning to accept modern medical health care, they still turn to indigenous health practitioners for most illnesses.

The national family planning programme entered this district in 1980 and introduced the contraceptive pill, the condom and the intra-uterine device (IUD). For most Sasak women the IUD is not an acceptable contraceptive because they feel too shy to expose their private parts to a doctor or nurse. Their husbands also won't allow this because, as they say, "If I, your husband have never seen you, surely somebody else is not allowed to see you!". Intercourse and childbirth occur under the *kain*, the cloth women wear.

Norplant was introduced in 1986 and 1987 as an alternative to the IUD because it is a long-lasting contraceptive. Current government policy is to strongly promote long-term methods. In Bayan this policy is translated into turning pill users into Norplant users and offering the implant to new contraceptive users. There is a strong emphasis on Norplant, which is promoted as the safest method of contraception.

The December 1990 report from the Bayan family planning team lists 1356 Norplant users, 520 IUD users, 3272 pill users, 386 injectable contraceptive users, 2 condom users and 160 people who have been sterilised. The district population is 42,208, with an estimated 6671 couples eligible for family planning, of which 85.38% "officially" practice family planning.

All couples who practice family planning are given a family planning card. The colour of the card refers to the kind of family planning service the clients choose. People receive a card if they participate actively in the family planning programme, irrespective of which method they choose. The red card refers to the government programme, which is fully subsidised. The white with blue card refers to the KB Mandiri, a programme which encourages the clients to pay for the contraceptives and services to some extent or in full.

A new policy adopted by the local government is that couples of reproductive age need to have a family planning card if they want an official letter from the local government. This group is called PUS, *pasangan usia subur*, couples who are in their fertile years and have one, two or more children. An official letter from the government is needed if a person wants to sell or buy land, to get a bank loan, to get permission to organised circumcision, hair cutting rituals and important events (*begawe adat*) related to the *adat*. In order to obtain the official letter, couples of reproductive age need to show their family planning card. This kind of measure is not limited to the family planning programme. Farmers are also required to be members of the government-organised farmers' cooperative and must show their membership card to obtain the letter from the government in the situations listed above. There are special programmes with an integrated approach which includes family planning. A team consisting of several departments, like agriculture, religious affairs and general health, visit a target area to give a two-day information course to the people about all the government programmes, including family planning. Family planning services are then carried out on the spot.

Participants in the study

Between September 1990 and February 1991, 65 women from three villages were interviewed about their experiences with contraceptives, menstruation and knowledge of traditional medicines. Five husbands were interviewed separately and a number of others participated during their wives' interviews. Ten traditional midwives and 13 other knowledgeable people were interviewed. Several of the latter were also Norplant users and were therefore also interviewed in that capacity. The interviews generally took place on the *barugaq*, a raised platform in front of the house on which all social events take place. This meant that very intimate questions were often difficult to ask. On the other hand, sometimes the interviews created discussions and more people contributed to the questions. Informal talks and participant observation were also used to gather information.[2]

Of the 65 women who were interviewed, 45 had used Norplant, from between one day to three years. Three of the women had just had the contraceptive implanted. Of the remaining 42 women with Norplant, 14 women had experienced no side-effects or side-effects that lasted less than three months. Eight women experienced amenorrhoea and 20 women experienced other disturbances in their bleeding pattern (see fig. 1). Apart from menstrual problems, other side-effects mentioned were: headaches, dizziness, vomiting, low energy (*kurang tenaga*), weight loss, weight gain, depression and loss of sexual drive. Three women had already had the implant removed and one had plans to have it removed because she had lost one capsule and suffered severe side-effects.

2 Participant observation is an anthropological method in which research is carried out by taking part in daily life.

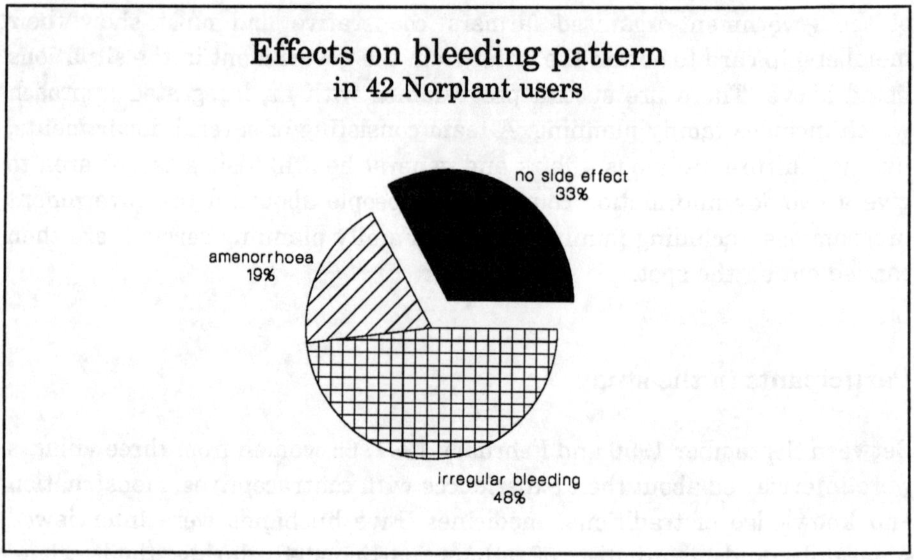

Figure 1

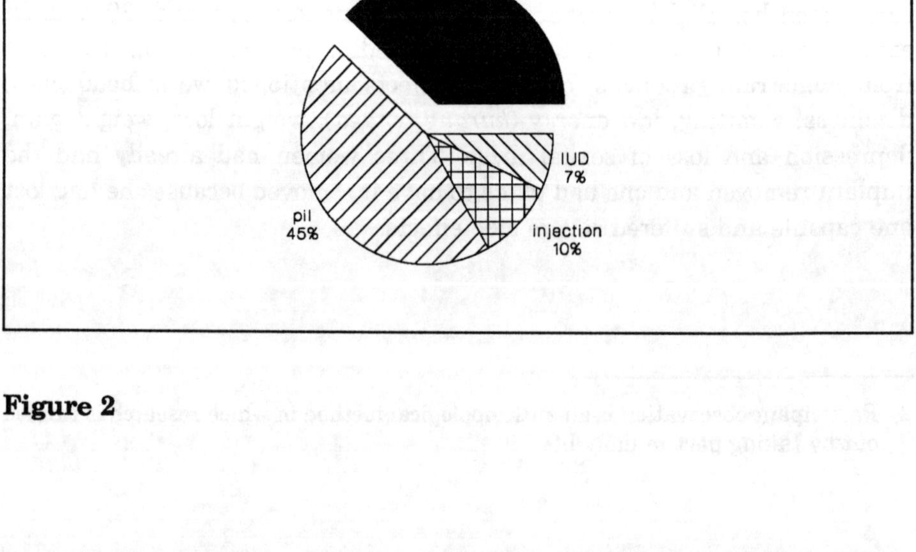

Figure 2

Twenty-six of these women had used another contraceptive previously (see fig. 2). Nineteen had used the contraceptive pill, four had used an injectable contraceptive and three had used an intra-uterine device (IUD). The majority of these women said that they had changed contraceptives because of side-effects, although a few said that they were also ordered to do so by the head of the hamlet or the doctor.

Two of the 19 women who had used the pill before the implant said that they had been happy with the pill and that they had changed because they were ordered to do so.

All of the women claimed that their menstruation was regular before the use of the implant. Although many women experienced side-effects, most said they were happy with the implant and that they would use it again after the expiration of the first set. Ten women expressed a wish for another child.

Attitudes towards menstruation

Quite a large number of women (28 out of 45) experienced changes in their menstrual cycle. What does this mean to these women? In the interviews, the following perspectives on the meaning of menstruation for Sasak women came up.

In the first place, they view it as something natural. It is considered a sign of good health if the menstrual flow is quick and not too heavy. It is not a healthy sign if it comes out slowly. The traditional medicines against menstrual pain are not widely used. Women worry about spilling blood and are careful that it does not show. They normally use underpants (up to five at a time), occasionally an old cloth or purchased menstrual pads if the flow is heavy.

Menstruation is also a powerful concept connected with their sense of womanhood, fertility and nature. In Bayan the women observe the regulations prescribed by Islam, like not being allowed to pray, to fast or to enter the mosque during menstruation. Women are also not allowed to have intercourse or to wash their hair during menstruation and they must take a ritual bath afterwards.

Besides the observance of Islamic regulations, there are taboos which are connected with the Wetu Telu *adat*. The perpetuating cycle of nature and seeds, growth and birth are central to traditional beliefs. The menstrual period is part of this cycle. During menstruation, the woman is considered unclean. Some women said that the black colour of the blood and the occasionally foul smell were proof of this. During her period the woman is not allowed to carry out duties related to the *adat*, such as attending and working on *adat* ceremonies and funerals. However, there was disagreement about whether menstruating women are not allowed to go to funerals or only not allowed to wash and touch the deceased, which is normally a woman's privilege. They are not allowed to fetch the rice from the rice barn and to plant or enter fields with special crops, like *lombok* (pepper), which are believed to wither if a menstruating woman enters the field. Rice planting is no problem, because the rice is cleaned in several rituals before it is stored in the rice barn.

Women tend to share their experiences with menstruation, especially the first menstruation, with others in their peer group. Most women felt too shy to tell their parents that their menses had begun. For some, telling their parents meant that they had to be purified by a religious leader. They experienced this as a kind of burden or punishment and tried to avoid it. The first menstruation is a time in which the girl is very susceptible to bad forces, and the first menstrual blood can be used as a tool in black magic. In former days a girl was not allowed to leave the house for a month when she menstruated for the first time.

Some health and field workers said that it was difficult to obtain correct information about menstruation from women in order to estimate whether a woman could be pregnant or not, because women were reluctant to talk about it. In the interviews, however, the women said that they felt free to talk about menstruation, especially between women, in private. In any other situation they would feel shy. To talk about pregnancy was sometimes less safe and they were careful not to mention how many months they were pregnant, because they believed that sometimes other people could hurt the baby if they knew.

During his wife's pregnancy, a man is not allowed to cut his hair or fingernails or to build anything which requires making knots or using a hammer and nails. These actions are considered to harm the child and to obstruct childbirth. These kinds of regulations for the husband do not exist during menstruation, except that intercourse is not allowed.

The respondents were adamant that intercourse did not take place during menstruation. They reacted with abhorrence at the suggestion that it probably sometimes "just happens". Not only is it forbidden by Islam, but it also could hurt the baby in the woman's womb. This belief corresponded to a view of menstruation as linked to potential pregnancy. A man could lose the spiritual power to say a *mantra*, a magic formula which is used to protect and clean the rice, among other things. Intercourse during menstruation is considered unhealthy for both the woman and the man.

Menstrual disturbances

What do menstrual disturbances mean to women in Bayan who use Norplant?

If they have no menstruation, women worry about a possible pregnancy or about the unclean blood which is not expelled from their bodies. They are afraid that the unclean blood will make them ill. If the health worker assures them that they are not pregnant and that lack of menstruation is not a health danger, the women appear to accept this and not to worry any more. However, one village health worker said that several women using Norplant asked him for medicines to induce menstruation.

If menstruation is long, heavy or very irregular, like five months without bleeding and then very heavy bleeding twice a month, women worry about their health. They are sometimes afraid they will have no blood left and may die. They feel that the blood takes away energy. These women visit health workers more often.

Regular but more frequent bleeding (for instance, twice a month) is accepted better than irregular bleeding.

The women did not discuss the effects of Norplant on their personal lives during the interviews. However, taking into consideration the regulations and taboos women face when they are menstruating, prolonged or frequent bleeding can influence women's social and personal lives. It can affect their relationships with their husbands because sexual intercourse is not allowed. Women can only do certain types of work in the fields and cannot take part in the traditional *adat* celebrations. These *adat* celebrations are generally held during special periods and play an important role in reinforcing social and family ties and obligations for mutual help. If a woman is unable to attend these gatherings for a longer time it could harm her position in society.

Prolonged bleeding may also have a psychological effect on a woman. The feeling that one is constantly unclean, that life-energy is being lost, can have a significant impact on a woman's sense of well-being.

The practical side should be considered as well. A woman with heavy or prolonged bleeding needs many pairs of underpants or has to buy expensive menstrual pads. These pads are sometimes difficult to throw away without people noticing. In one part of the district, women live seven kilometres from a water source. The water is carried on horseback and motorcycles to the villages. In these circumstances it is very difficult for women to wash themselves and their clothing frequently.

Many women mentioned bleeding problems during the interviews, but they didn't complain about not being able to attend ceremonies or perform duties which are not allowed during menstruation. This was sometimes mentioned to health workers, however. Women felt embarrassed to talk about not being able to have intercourse, especially when the interview situation was less private. With regard to other side-effects which some of the women experienced, the women who said that they had "less energy" did complain that they couldn't work as hard as usual. As in many developing countries, it is very important for women in Bayan to be able to work hard. Their social esteem and direct survival partially depend on it.

Help-seeking behaviour

It was expected that women who suffered from menstrual disturbances or other side-effects would not only seek advice from a medical health worker, but would also try self-medication or help from a traditional healer. This appeared not to be the case.

According to the women interviewed, the menstrual disturbances and other side-effects they experienced were caused by the contraceptive. They saw no reason to go to a traditional healer for the side-effects. They distinguished clearly between health problems they thought were caused by the implant and other illnesses. They didn't use home-made *jamu's* (medicinal herbal tonics) or medicines which they bought themselves. This did not apply to problems they did not directly relate to the implant, like depression.

If they had complaints, more than half of the women went to the clinic or health post for help and advice. One woman said that she didn't go to the doctor because she couldn't afford to.

This was confirmed by the traditional midwives. They said that they could not treat menstrual disturbances caused by contraceptives. They always send those patients to the clinic. Only one male *dukun* (indigenous medical practitioner) who helped as a birth attendant said that he treated a woman with heavy bleeding. According to him, this heavy bleeding could not be caused by a device implanted in the arm. How could it possibly influence a woman's womb? He therefore treated her and was successful, he said.

Contacts with health workers

The health workers interviewed included the doctor, one clinic and two sub-clinic level nurses, one midwife, the head of the family planning programme and a family planning field worker.

The women who went to the clinic or health post with bleeding disturbances were often told that these were only normal side-effects and not a problem (*effek sampingan yang biasa dan tidak apa-apa*). Health workers stated that bleeding problems can be treated, although not always successfully. Amenorrhoea from Norplant is not considered to be treatable. Instead, health workers counselled women with amenorrhoea to reassure them that this was not a sign of pregnancy or bad health.

Health workers said that women often came with complaints which they blamed on the implant, although the implant was not always the cause of the problem. They said, "They blame everything on the implant, even if they have a fever". On the other hand, not all health workers were well informed about potential side-effects from Norplant.

A discussion was recorded between a health worker, in this case the *mantri* (a male nurse on a village subclinic level) and a prospective Norplant user. The woman asked whether the implant could be removed if she had side-effects like bleeding. She had heard that the doctor made it very difficult for users to get the implant removed. The *mantri* agreed, explaining that the government would suffer a financial loss if they removed an implant, and stated that the only side-effects from Norplant were disturbances in the menstrual cycle.

The woman asked, "What if I am going to die?".

"Nobody ever dies from the implant," the *mantri* said. "There are only bleeding problems."

After some discussion, the *mantri* agreed that headaches could also possibly be a side-effect of the implant, but this was very difficult to determine, as many people suffered from headaches in this area. The *mantri* said that he was never properly trained or taught about Norplant. He didn't know much about it. The only thing he knew was that he could treat bleeding problems with vitamin K. Sometimes the bleeding stopped; sometimes it didn't. He didn't know why. He only assisted the family planning worker with the programme. If the bleeding problems persisted, he would refer the woman to the doctor, who treated her with oestrogen (Lynoral – ethinyloestradiol 0.05 mg).

This conversation shows that it is sometimes difficult for women to obtain correct information or recognition of side-effects which might occur when using the implant. The *mantri*, one of the first health workers people turn to, was not properly trained in this case. This *mantri* felt that problems which arise out of the use of contraceptives should be the responsibility of the family planning programme. He did not see them as general health problems. The lack of proper training and the division of perceived responsibilities between health workers and family planning workers are also discussed by Ward et al. (1990) and in the report by the YKB (1986). Health workers feel responsible for health screening and medical procedures and family planning field workers are held responsible for dissemination of information and for follow-up. But, "...(family planning) field workers generally do not have adequate information and background in Norplant to feel comfortable about advising clients in the management of side-effects" (Ward et al. 1990, pp. 48-49).

The topic of more emotional side-effects was addressed in an interview with the physician and a nurse. When asked about the occurrence of side-effects like depression or loss of sexual drive, they said that they had never heard a woman mention these side-effects. But, they confessed, they also never asked about these problems. During the interviews two women mentioned depression and loss of sexual drive, but only after they were asked about these problems. This does not mean that they suffered side-effects from the implant, but it is a possibility which should not be ignored. In Bayan sexual matters are considered private. Health workers and clients do not talk freely about sex. Women mention instead that they cannot perform daily prayers because of frequent bleeding, which is a more acceptable problem. *Kurang tenaga*, lower energy, is treated as a physical problem, although it may be a sign of emotional disturbances.

In general, common side-effects like menstrual disturbances or dizziness are recognized by health workers. However, the training and education of health workers determine the extent to which they are able to recognize other side-effects which appear less often.

Many women may not be questioned thoroughly about their health concerns, partly due to lack of knowledge, time or skills, and partly perhaps because even if health workers were to ask about all possible side-effects, they wouldn't know how to deal with them.

Health workers are under a lot of pressure to keep Norplant users from deciding to remove the implant. Only the doctor is authorised to decide about a removal. Between June 1989 and February 1991, the implant was only removed before the period of effectiveness was over in 17 cases out of a total of 1356 implant users in Bayan (1.25% of users). It was not possible to obtain full information on the reasons for the removals, as only carbon copies of records were available and not all were legible. However, some of the reasons for removals were side-effects, pregnancy and a desire for another child.

Women often mentioned that they felt put off when they were repeatedly told that their health problems were normal and not a matter for concern.

It is obvious that there are no criteria which are clear to users to estimate the seriousness of side-effects. They may consider a side-effect to be serious but are told by health workers that it is "just normal, no problem". The health worker determines what is normal. The same is true for what is acceptable or not acceptable. Some women said that they first expected that the implant be removed because it was not suitable or "did not agree" with them (*implant tidak cocok sama saya*). Instead they were told that their problem was normal. Some still suffer from bleeding or other side-effects.

Information given to users

The information given to women is in general limited. The most important messages are that Norplant is the safest method, that it is effective for five years and that it cannot be removed before that time. Sometimes women are told that if there is no menstruation the implant is suitable for the user, but if there is irregular bleeding they should come to the clinic. No written materials are used. Although every packaged set of Norplant capsules contains user information and instructions, these are never handed out. Health and field workers say that this is because the people are too backward with regard to modern medical care and would not understand the package inserts.

Volunteers from the women's welfare movement (PKK) and community health posts (Posyandu) are trained and given information about contraceptives, so that they can pass the information on to friends and fellow villagers. The same is true for local leaders. But, as the head of one hamlet said, "I cannot remember it properly. Yes, I have been trained, but it was some time ago." These people must inform and recruit prospective Norplant users when a family planning session is scheduled. One women said that the hamlet head threatened her with the police; another women said that he told her, "If the pill agrees with you (*cocok*), the implant will agree with you", and ordered her to change contraceptives. Unfortunately, she had problems with the implant and had to have it removed. But she suffered for two years with severe side-effects before she dared to ask for the implant's removal. By then she felt so ill and angry that she refused to take no for an answer and demanded that the implant be removed.

These might be isolated incidents. It is not official Indonesian government policy to force people to use contraceptives. However, the top-down system of setting targets which eventually must be reached by local leaders can lead to these sorts of situations. Some local leaders turn to enforcement instead of giving information.

This problem extends beyond the local leaders. As one family planning worker said:

> "There is a difference in education. People with secondary school education understand what we are trying to explain when we speak about the programme and contraceptives. But people without education do not understand. And then the element of pressure comes in. People with a low education need an example. If they see that a friend is satisfied with the implant, they want one too."

Another family planning worker explained the use of pressure this way:

> "If the target is still high and has not yet been reached and the people are difficult to reach, the army makes them a little bit afraid so that they are willing to come together for a family planning session."

In the 1990 report by Ward et al., these problems of "persuasion" by family planning workers are discussed in the context that field workers do not have proper training in counselling. They reported that field workers expressed interest in learning more about counselling because they thought it would help them in their work.

The concept of counselling is based on providing a range of information, including alternative options, to the client. There should be two-way communication. In Indonesia, this is constrained by several factors. One is the authoritarian nature of the government and the social structure. This is reflected in the way social programmes are carried out, no matter how well-designed and well-meaning these programmes may be (Hull 1991, p. 6). The existence of targets which are not set locally means that those who carry out family planning programmes are afraid that if people are given too much information or too much room to think for themselves, they will not accept the contraceptive the government wants them to use.

A discussion which illustrates this was recorded on a field visit with a representative of the women's welfare movement (PKK) and several wives of government officials. They wanted to register the prospective family planning acceptors in a particular hamlet[3]. One of the hamlet women said that she wanted to try the pill first. She said that if the pill didn't agree with her, she could stop. All the officials' wives tried to convince her that she should use the implant, stating that the pill had many more side-effects than the implant. In the end they almost implied that the pill was bad for her health. They felt so pressured to promote Norplant that they did not give correct information and discredited the oral contraceptive.

During an interview it was sometimes difficult to obtain an answer if a woman was asked what she would like to know about Norplant. Women are not used to being asked their opinion. Sometimes they replied only after several other questions had passed. Some questions were: "What happens with the dirty blood that doesn't come out? What happens if I lose too much blood? How much does removal cost?"

Removal on request

It is very difficult for women to get their implant removed before the five-year period of efficacy is over. The normal procedure, except if a woman is pregnant, is to try to solve the problem first with medication. If this doesn't help and the woman has already gone to the clinic several times, removal will be considered. According to the doctor, if a woman really insists on removal, he cannot refuse it because she chose the implant of her own free will. However, he will often try to talk the woman out of it.

One woman went to the clinic to ask for removal because she was divorced and no longer had a husband. She was told that if she had no side-effects it was better to keep the implant in. Although this is not an official policy, it might be interpreted as such at a local level. A few findings from the study conducted by Ward et al. (1990) confirm this. With respect to the issue of removal on demand, Ward, et al. report that people are expected to keep the implants for the entire five year efficacy period. One family planning programme manager interviewed said, "If they request removal, they are reminded that they gave their word." Ward, et al. also expressed concerns that the family planning programme has not yet trained enough people to remove Norplant.

3 Volunteers provide information and encourage couples to accept the family planning programme and to use contraceptives. Wives of government officials are expected to do their share in this promotional work.

Often, however, women do not dare to ask for removal because of side-effects or because they wish for a new child. They are afraid that they will be refused. One of the women said that she had heard that the doctor would say, "If I remove it for you, all the other women will come as well to get it removed." Whether or not these stories are true, they keep women from asking for removal.

Other obstacles are fear of the removal operation and the cost of removal, which was 10,000 rupiahs at the time of the study. This is approximately US $5 or the equivalent of three to six days' wages for working in the fields. In July 1992, the cost of removal was increased to 25,000 rupiahs if the woman wanted Norplant removed before five years and if she was not suffering from severe side-effects. Family planning and health workers said that this measure was designed to prevent women's friends from also coming to the clinic and asking for removal of the implant.

Sometimes women keep Norplant because they see no alternative. One woman suffered from severe bleeding problems but didn't dare ask for removal because she had tried the pill, which gave her headaches. She was afraid of the IUD and saw no acceptable alternative to the implant.

Although many problems have been discussed here, it should be emphasised that all the people interviewed spoke well of the health workers. They said that the health workers were kind to them and that they were always prepared to help them. The health workers expressed real concern for the people and spoke their local language. They would often wear casual clothes when they went into the field in order not to frighten people with their uniforms. There were occasions when people could not pay for medicines and were told they could pay less or even later. The Bayan people felt that the health workers were there for them.

The interviewees were less clear about the family planning workers. Some said that they did not know the family planning workers well enough to voice an opinion about them. One family planning worker who had lived in the region for 10 years was well liked.

Many women talked about the problems they experienced with Norplant, but most of the users were content with the implant. Even those who said that they were pressured into using the implant stated that they felt good about the method. Women who experienced side-effects also considered the implant to be safe. They felt that they didn't have to worry about it because it was always in their arm. An occasional ambivalence could be detected in these positive attitudes towards the implant. Although some women said they were content with the implant, they kept asking whether nothing could be done about menstrual problems and whether it was not bad for their health. The large number of women who already use the implant in this area plays an important role in user satisfaction. On several occasions women were heard urging their friends to use the implant.

The people of Bayan are aware of the benefits of family planning. Many young mothers said they were happy with only two children. They said that it was much better for the children and they were not as busy and could do more work in the fields.

Conclusion

The focus of this study was on the experiences of women with Norplant. Although the study was conducted over a relatively short time period and covered a small area of Lombok, a few themes can be abstracted.

The information given to women about Norplant is in general limited and emphasises the implant's positive aspects. Health and family planning workers are either afraid that women will refrain from using the implant if informed about the possible side-effects, other than menstrual disturbances, or assume that the women would not understand more extensive information. Women are also given information about the implant by volunteers who, although formally trained, often cannot offer balanced information on various other contraceptive methods.

Lack of privacy is often a reason not to discuss more sensitive problems with the health workers. Social and cultural constraints prevent users and health workers from discussing, for example, the influence of Norplant on their sexual lives and daily well-being.

The implications of menstrual disturbances or other side-effects of Norplant are significant. Women worry about how the side-effects will affect their health. Their social and sexual life can be adversely influenced by, for example, bleeding problems. Women in this and other studies conducted in Indonesia (Poernomo Sigit Sidi 1990; Ward et al. 1990), however, do not complain about the implications of Norplant use on their general well-being. In the words of Ward et al. "There is a tradition in Indonesia of individual views being of less significance than those of important reference groups. Women who are part of this tradition are likely to accept a contraceptive method because it is a decision made for them by an important reference group. The use of Norplant is often promoted by powerful groups representing government, religious, or military organisations." (1990, p. 31-32).

Not only do important reference groups set the standards on how Norplant should be viewed, but the medical establishment and the family planning programme set the standards for what complaints about Norplant use are acceptable. The women, the users, have to move within these dominant views on Norplant. They do not have access to adequate and balanced information. Their complaints about side-effects are often not accepted by the health workers as valid. They cannot easily change contraceptive methods when they want to.

The top-down model of the family planning programme and the extensive use of targetting creates room for possible coercive pressure on women to use Norplant. Although this might not be the official policy of the Indonesian government, there are few control mechanisms to prevent these potentially abusive actions.

Several of the statements of family planning workers and Norplant users interviewed in this study are disturbing, for example: reliance on the army to "make people a little afraid" so they attend a family planning session; several Norplant users' assertions that they were ordered to use Norplant instead of the pill; and artificially high prices for removal to discourage "unnecessary" early removals. If these statements are accurate, they are clear infringements of human rights.

The acceptability of Norplant needs to be seen within the social, political and cultural context in which it is used. Within a political context of potential coercion, the appropriateness of Norplant, or any other contraceptive technology which women cannot choose to start or stop using at will, can be seriously questioned.

Indonesia currently has more Norplant users than any other country in the world. How many Indonesian Norplant users find that their daily well-being is improved because they use Norplant, a highly effective contraceptive? How many would choose to have it removed if it was as easy to get rid of Norplant as it is to obtain it? These questions cannot be answered by the current study. However, this study does raise the need to address issues of contraceptive choice, removal on demand, the effects of menstrual disturbances on day-to-day life and the need for appropriate information and counselling. Women need to be properly informed and given genuine choices. Only then can they use birth control to exercise their right to determine their own family size.

References

Affandi B. *Clinical, Pharmacological and Epidemiological Studies on a Levonorgestrel Implant Contraceptive.* [Dissertation]. Jakarta: University of Indonesia, 1987.

Affandi B. "Norplant Introduction in Indonesia." Workshop on Implementation of Large Scale Norplant Programmes Subsequent to Pre-introduction/Clinical Trial

Phase: JHPIEGO, Klinik Raden Saleh and BKKBN, Jakarta, Indonesia, 10-14 December 1990.

Affandi B., Prihartono J., Lubis F., Sutedi H., Samil RS. "Insertion and Removal of Norplant Contraceptive Implants by Physicians and Non-physicians in an Indonesian Clinic." *Studies in Family Planning* 1987; 18(5):302-305.

Hull T.H. "Reports of Coercion in the Indonesian Vasectomy Program." Confidential Report to AIDAB, 1991.

Lubis F., Prihartono J., Agoestina T., Affandi B., Sutedi H. "One-Year Experience with Norplant Implants in Indonesia." *Studies in Family Planning* 1983; 14 (6/7):181-184.

Poernomo Sigit Sidi I. "Report on the Use of Norplant in Family Planning, Indonesia." Symposium on Long-Acting Hormonal Contraceptives, Madrid, 1989.

Poernomo Sigit Sidi I. *Improving Norplant Service Providers' Counselling Skills in Indonesia*. Indonesia: Yayasan Kusuma Buana and PATH, 1990.

Prihartono J. "Factors Associated with Due and Overdue Five Year Removal." *Norplant Removal Study*. Indonesia: Yayasan Kusuma Buana and The Population Council, 1990.

Sutedi H., Affandi B., Prihartono J., Lubis F. "Introduction of the Norplant Subdermal Contraceptive System into a Family Planning Programme." Indonesia: Yayasan Kusuma Buana, (n.d.).

Ward J.S., Poernomo Sigit Sidi I, Simmons R., Simmons G.B. "Service Delivery Systems and Quality of Care in the Implementation of Norplant in Indonesia". Unpublished report. New York: The Population Council, 1990.

Warwick D.P. "The Indonesian Family Planning Program: Government Influence and Client Choice." *Population and Development Review* 1986; (12):3.

Yayasan Kusuma Buana. *Norplant Acceptability Study*. Jakarta, Indonesia, 1986.

Yayasan Kusuma Buana. *Hasil Penelitian Manajemen Norplant (Action Based Norplant Research) 1987-1988*. Indonesia: Badan Koordinasi Keluarga Berencana Nasional dan Yayasan Kusuma Buana.

Zimmerman, M., Haffey J., Crane E., Szumowski D., Alvarez F., Bhiromrut P., Brache V., Lubis F, Salah M., Shaaban M., Sawky B., Poernomo Sigit Sidi I. "Assessing the Acceptability of Norplant Implants in Four Countries: Findings from Focus Group Research." *Studies in Family Planning* 1990; 21 (2):92-103.

Experience of Norplant by Finnish family planning practitioners

by Eeva Ollila, Kristiina Kajesalo and Elina Hemminki

Introduction

Finland is the country which manufactures Norplant and one of the few industrialised countries using it. The Finnish experience with Norplant may therefore be of interest both within industrialised and non-industrialised countries.

Finland was the first country to allow registration and marketing of the implantable contraceptive Norplant. It was registered at the end of 1983 and appeared on the market in 1984. At first only gynaecologists were allowed to prescribe Norplant, but since 1985 it can be prescribed by any physician. Norplant-2, a two-rod modification which is effective for three years, was registered in Finland in 1986 and is still not registered in any other country. A Finnish company, Leiras Pharmaceuticals, is the sole producer of both Norplant and Norplant-2. Leiras also has a monopoly over marketing in all countries except the United States, where Norplant is marketed by Wyeth, and the UK, where it is marketed by Roussel.

This study is based on interviews with family planning practitioners in Finland. It describes their experiences with Norplant and attitudes towards it. A literature search on Norplant in Finnish medical journals was also conducted in order to gain an overview of the literature available to Finnish physicians.

The interviews took place in the fall of 1989 and the spring of 1990. Norplant had then been on the market for about six years in Finland.

Family planning services in Finland

The population of Finland is about five million people. Contraception is widely used (Haddad et al. 1984). In 1987 an estimated 65% of women of reproductive age used contraceptives. Of these, 25% used intrauterine devices (IUDs), 18% used oral contraceptives and 20% used barrier methods. An estimated 1% of women of reproductive age use Norplant (Makkonen and Hemminki 1991).

Family planning services are provided in the public sector by health centres and hospital outpatient clinics and in the private sector by private practitioners. Condoms and spermicides can be obtained without a prescription.

Public primary health care services are divided administratively into 213 health centres. All of these centres have sufficient facilities for minor surgical procedures. All public health centres have also been required by law since 1975 to provide family planning services (Vienonen 1987). Approximately one third of women of reproductive age obtain family planning services from public health centres (Kivijärvi 1987). Norplant is mainly used in the public sector, according to one of the two medical representatives for Norplant in Finland (Syrjä, personal communication, 29 Sept. 1989).

Interviews of family planning physicians

Physicians with experience with Norplant and a small stratified random sample of family planning practitioners were selected for interviews.

We randomly chose one urban and one rural health centre from each of the 11 counties in continental Finland. The names of the 213 health centres in Finland, categorised by county and urban or rural status, were set in boxes and one name was blindly drawn from each grouping. Each of these health centres was contacted by telephone to identify the physician in charge of family planning services. In two health centres where a nurse, rather than a physician, was responsible for coordinating family planning services, we interviewed the coordinating nurse. The 20 physicians (see Table 1,I) and two nurses were sent a letter briefly describing the survey and its purpose. They were then interviewed by telephone. Those who had inserted at least one set of Norplant rods were classified as providers (see Table 1,IA), and those who had never inserted Norplant as non-providers. This classification also reflected the policy of all the health centres concerned. One doctor refused the interview, saying that he had never provided Norplant and had nothing to say about the method. He is retained in the survey as a non-provider. The two nurses are included as non-providers because no one in their health centres inserted Norplant.

Interviews were structured informally with a check list of open-ended questions. Different questions were used for providers and non-providers (see Appendix 1 for a list of these questions). Each interview lasted between 20 to 30 minutes. The answers were written down during the interview.

We also interviewed family planning practitioners known to have experience with Norplant. They were chosen because of their expertise with Norplant and are referred to as experts in the following text (see Table 1,II). This group included seven gynaecologists, one general practitioner and one nurse working in five big family planning centres or hospital outpatient clinics in the Helsinki area and two general practitioners from health centres outside the Helsinki area. Four of the experts had been associated with the development of Norplant, three of whom were working in the same family planning unit.

The expert interviews were not structured. They lasted for approximately one hour. We interviewed those in Helsinki in person and those outside the Helsinki area by telephone. Notes were made during the interviews and a more detailed account was written later.

All of the interviews were conducted by one of the authors. The interviews were conducted in an informal manner, aimed at an open discussion between colleagues, and so were not structured strictly or recorded. Because of the informal nature of the interviews, the data from some physicians was incomplete.

Provision or non-provision of Norplant

Of the 22 practitioners in the random sample, only 10 had inserted Norplant. As shown in Table 1, the amount of experience with Norplant was low among these 10 physicians. Most had inserted Norplant in 10 or fewer women. No difference was found between urban and rural communities.

Table 1 Distribution of physicians by their reported number of insertions and removals of Norplant

	Whole random sample N=20[1]		Providers N=10		Experts N=10[2]	
	I		IA		II	
	insertions	removals	insertions	removals	insertions	removals
0	10	8	0	1	0	0
1-5	2	11	2	8	0	1
6-10	6	0	6	0	0	2
11-20	2	0	2	0	1	4
21-49	0	0	0	0	5	0
50-	0	1	0	1	2	1
No information	0	0	0	0	2	2

[1] The two nurses working in non-providing health centres are excluded, because insertions and removals are only done by physicians.
[2] The nurse interviewed is excluded.

Interviews with practitioners providing Norplant

The following information was provided by the 10 Norplant providers in the random sample and the 11 experts who were interviewed.

Norplant and Norplant-2: The relative popularity of these two forms of Norplant varied. Some practitioners preferred Norplant-2 because there are fewer rods to be inserted or removed and because of the shorter period of use. On the other hand, in one big family planning clinic where both forms of Norplant have been researched, Norplant-2 is not inserted any more because the rods tend to break on removal. Other practitioners also mentioned the tendency for Norplant-2 rods to break as the reason they prefer Norplant.

Information: When asked where women get their information on Norplant, the providers often said that it was from lay sources such as women's magazines (n=6), the mass media in general (n=1), or friends (n=3). Only two mentioned health professionals. Five of the nine experts who were asked this question considered women's magazines an important source of information, but six of them also said that either they or other health professionals were important sources of information. Many practitioners believed that women's magazines and the mass media in general gave information on Norplant which was too optimistic. As one provider said, "Women get their information from the mass media. They have lots of wrong ideas about the implant. They presume that it is a super-method, easy to use and without side-effects."

The practitioners themselves had received their information mainly from the manufacturer and, to a lesser extent, from colleagues and medical journals.

Selection of users: When asked how they selected the women to whom they would recommend Norplant, five of the 10 providers answered that they themselves did not recommend it to anyone. One other provider said that "the women request it more than I insert it". The experts were not asked this question, but four of them mentioned during discussion that they would recommend Norplant to some restricted target groups.

All of the practitioners said it was important to select Norplant users carefully. Women's expectations were reported to influence the decision, but no one recommended Norplant as a method of first choice. However, one expert saw it as an alternative to the IUD for women over 35. Usually Norplant was prescribed only after other methods, such as oral contraceptives containing oestrogens and IUD's, had been found to be unsuitable. This was stated by seven of the 10 providers, and by eight of the 11 experts. Some also mentioned women who had completed their families and did not want to be sterilised or were waiting before being sterilised as possible users.

A special user group, "asocial women", was mentioned by four of the 10 providers. An additional two had each once given Norplant to alcoholic women with mental problems. Five of the 11 experts mentioned asocial women as one target group for Norplant. Five of the practitioners defined "asocial women" as women who did not remember or were unable to take their oral contraceptives regularly. The others also specified alcoholics, women with psychiatric problems, women with several induced abortions, or women who had removed their IUDs themselves.

A definite need for long-term contraception lasting three to five years was spontaneously mentioned as a precondition for a Norplant insertion by four providers and five experts. The long period of effectiveness was considered a limiting factor in the use of Norplant because the "moods of Finnish women change quickly", as one practitioner put it.

The eight providers and six experts who were asked about prior counselling considered it crucial. Counselling consisted of information about the long-term contraceptive effectiveness of the implants, the operational nature of insertion and removal and the possibility of menstrual irregularities. Three providers and three experts used counselling to discourage women from using the method. This was expressed most strongly by one expert with a lot of experience with Norplant: "50% of the women who have a fixed idea that they want Norplant will change their minds when they are told about the bleeding irregularities and the minor surgical operations associated with the method."

There are no official recommendations about prescribing progestin-only oral contraceptives (mini-pills) to assess Norplant's suitability. However, we learned about this practice during one of the early interviews and asked about it in all of the remaining interviews.

All of the seven providers who were asked about prescribing mini-pills said that they prescribe them for a period of two to six months before making a final decision about Norplant insertion. Three experts were asked whether they prescribed mini-pills prior to inserting Norplant. Two of the three also prescribed them.

The mini-pills were used mainly to test for bleeding irregularities. Practitioners also looked for other possible side-effects from progestins. The experience with the mini-pill was interpreted in two ways: to predict the quantity of side-effects a woman would develop and also the woman's tolerance towards the side-effects. The one expert who did not prescribe mini-pills prior to Norplant insertion said that there was no correlation between side-effects with mini-pills and Norplant.

Exclusion criteria: The providers and experts were asked to state their reasons for not providing Norplant (Table 2). The reasons varied, but many reflected an attempt to minimise problems with bleeding irregularities. Women with existing bleeding irregularities or low tolerance for such problems were not given Norplant. The practitioners had somewhat inconsistent criteria for age. Some did not provide Norplant to young women; others did not provide it to older women. One practitioner regarded women over 40 as a special target group. The contraindications listed in Pharmaca Fennica (see Box 1) were not usually mentioned by the practitioners.

Table 2 Criteria for not inserting Norplant

	Providers (N=10)	Experts (N=11)
Prior irregular bleeding	4	2
Intolerance towards bleeding irregularities	3	5
Heavy weight (>70 or >80 kg)	0	4[1]
Young women (<30 years)	3[2]	2
Older women who smoke (>35 or >40 years)	0	3[3]
History of thrombosis	0	2
Migraine	0	2
Other[4]	3	5

1 In addition, two experts would consider inserting Norplant also to heavier women, but would remove capsules after three years of use.
2 Includes young women with side-effects from oral contraceptives (one provider), and young women with prior bleeding irregularities (one provider). The latter were also listed under "prior irregular bleeding".
3 Includes women over 40 regardless of smoking status (one expert).
4 Includes nervousness, tendency to anaemia, acne, history of liver disease, epilepsy, hypertonia, premenstrual tension, weak motivation for contraception.

Side-effects: The providers and experts were asked what side-effects, if any, they had observed with Norplant use in their own practice. They were specifically asked about the occurrence of irregular bleeding and amenorrhoea (lack of menstrual bleeding). They were also asked an open question about observation of other side-effects.

Irregular bleeding was frequently observed. Estimates of the frequency of this problem ranged from under 50% to 100% (Table 3). Amenorrhoea was not found as commonly. Two experts estimated that its frequency was around 10%. The practitioners' view of the significance of amenorrhoea for women varied. Some believed that women were usually happy not to menstruate, but others thought that women found it disturbing.

Four providers and five experts said that they prescribed drugs to treat irregular bleeding. Progestins were most commonly prescribed, for a ten-day to a three-month period. Oral contraceptives containing oestrogens and progestins had also been prescribed for three months. One provider and one expert had used progestins to treat amenorrhoea and mentioned that the scheme for treating irregular bleeding with progestins was taught in an information session organised by the manufacturer of Norplant. Most practitioners who had treated bleeding irregularities with drugs would do so only rarely. Some said that the treatment was not very successful. Three experts did not approve of using oral hormones for either bleeding irregularities or amenorrhoea. One expert used treatment only for bleeding irregularities and one expert only for amenorrhoea.

Table 3 Observed side-effects[1] of Norplant

	Providers (N=10)	Experts (N=11)
Irregular bleeding	9	11
Amenorrhoea	5	7
Pregnancy	2	5
Acne	2	4
Weight gain	2	5
Bloating	2	1
Mood changes	1	5
Headaches and migraine	0	5
Other[2]	1	2

[1] Irregular bleeding and amenorrhoea were specifically asked about; others were spontaneous reports.
[2] Includes dizziness, leg cramps and ovarian cysts.

Reasons for discontinuing use: The reasons for discontinuing Norplant reported by providers and experts were similar to those mentioned as side-effects (Table 3). Overwhelmingly, the most frequent reason for discontinuing was irregular bleeding. Only one provider mentioned that amenorrhoea had led to early removal of Norplant. Additional infrequent reasons for removal of Norplant were visibility of the implant, ovarian cysts, thrombosis, breast cancer and leg cramps.

The rates of removal were recorded in one large family planning clinic in which 202 sets of Norplant were inserted during 1988 and 1989. By the end of 1989, after 0-2 years of use, one quarter (51) of these implants had already been removed. The reasons for discontinuation are given in Table 4. During 1990 and the first half of 1991 only 75 sets of Norplant were inserted in this clinic.

Table 4 Reasons for discontinuation of Norplant use in one family planning clinic

		Clinic I Years 1988-89 (N=51)
Wish to get pregnant		14%
Side-effects		80%
Bleeding irregularities	65%	
Psychological changes	6%	
Others[1]	9%	
Pregnancy		6%
Total		100%

[1] Including weight gain, swelling, acne, headaches and leg cramps.

In another large family planning clinic 195 sets of Norplant were inserted during 1988 and 1989. During the same period 261 sets were removed. In 82 cases (31%) the rods were removed because the period of effectiveness had expired and new sets were inserted. Women's reasons for discontinuing use were estimated to be similar to the ones presented in Table 4. Exact figures were not available, however.

The number of insertions of Norplant per year was declining in both of these clinics. Still, in the second clinic a noteworthy number of women decided to continue to use Norplant after their first set of implants had expired.

Pregnancies during Norplant use: The 10 providers had encountered six pregnancies during Norplant use among their patients. The experts knew of more pregnancies, but it was not clear how often the same patients were mentioned because most experts were working with a joint system of patient referrals.

The second family planning centre mentioned above also serves as a referral centre. They had encountered 22 pregnancies during Norplant use from 1983-1991. During 1988 and 1989 there were 13 pregnancies. In 20 of these 22 cases, Norplant with six rods had been used. The type of Norplant used is not recorded in the remaining two cases. Most pregnancies had occurred within the first three years of use. Four of the women used drugs for epilepsy and a few were overweight, but in most cases no factor was found which could explain the method failure. It is not possible to estimate the overall method failure rate from our study. However, the experts we interviewed estimated the efficacy of Norplant to be similar to the best oral contraceptives and IUDs.

Insertion and removal procedures: The providers and experts were asked about the duration of insertions and removals of Norplant and about any problems they encountered. All the providers regarded insertions as easy. The experts were somewhat more reserved. "Insertions are deceitfully easy," stated one expert. Another believed that only gynaecologists should insert Norplant. One expert had seen a case of massive bleeding associated with insertion and a case of local irritation at the site of insertion associated with a rod breaking. Another had heard of nerve injury during insertions.

Most insertion problems were discovered only when the implants were removed. The providers and experts had observed the following incorrect insertions: too deep (one provider and three experts); rods too widely spread (three providers and two experts); rods damaged during insertion, with the possible consequence of the hormone leaking out or breaking during removal (two providers, four experts). One provider and two experts suspected that rods had moved from the site of insertion. Many of the physicians also commented that removal was more difficult because of fibrous capsule formation around Norplant rods.

Removals were considered difficult or sometimes difficult by most providers and experts (Table 5). Even the experts who reported short average removal times had all encountered some difficult removals which had called for additional incisions or a second attempt. A rather common removal problem mentioned was that of rods breaking during removal (one provider and seven experts). The use of ultrasound to locate the rods was uncommon. Only two had heard of this being done. No one had used an x-ray for this purpose. Only one of the experts interviewed mentioned a referral of a difficult removal to his clinic.

Table 5 Removal of Norplant

	Providers (N=9)[1]	Experts (N=10)[2]
Average time		
< 20 min	4	6
> 20 min	5	3
no information	0	1
Procedure		
easy[3]	2	1
difficult[4]	7	9

[1] One had no experience of removals.
[2] Excluding the nurse.
[3] Includes "easy, but time consuming".
[4] Includes "sometimes difficult".

Interviews with non-providers

Out of the 22 practitioners working in health centres, 12 had never inserted Norplant. Reasons for not providing Norplant are presented in Table 6. Two health centres had previously had a physician who provided Norplant, but the current physician no longer provided it due to negative experiences, such as bleeding disorders and difficult removals. In one other health centre which had previously provided Norplant, the physician now in charge of family planning services still had a positive attitude towards Norplant, but had never recommended or inserted it during her two years at the clinic. Four non-providers mentioned that they could refer women to private practitioners or hospital outpatient clinics to obtain Norplant. Two of them would do so only if the woman insisted. The other two seemed to consider Norplant a method only to be provided by gynaecologists. Six non-providers had some patients who were Norplant users. The Norplant had either been inserted elsewhere or previously in the same health centre.

Table 6 Reasons for not providing Norplant

	Numbers[1] (N=12)
Characteristics of the implants[2]	7
No need for Norplant	7
Shortage of doctors or lack of hygienic facilities	3
No information	3

[1] Each practitioner could give several reasons.
[2] The most common responses were difficulties in removals and bleeding irregularities.

Review of Finnish medical literature on Norplant

This review was carried out in order to complement the survey and to gain an overview of published Finnish medical opinion on Norplant.

The entry in the Finnish prescription guide Pharmaca Fennica is listed in full in Box 1. The entry in the guide is provided by the manufacturer, but is based on text approved by the Finnish drug control authorities during registration.

We also conducted a literature search on Norplant using FINMED, which covers Finnish medical journals, to find out what recommendations were being made for Norplant use in Finland. We accepted only articles published in national non-commercial medical journals. The words contraception, contraceptives, contraceptive agents, and contraceptive devices were used as key words and all the articles were read to find those which mentioned Norplant.

Fourteen articles with information on Norplant were published between 1980 and 1990, of which three were solely on Norplant (Holma 1984; Holma 1987; Toivonen 1985). The remaining eleven articles cover various aspects of contraception and mention Norplant among other methods (Erkkola 1983; Haukkamaa 1987; Heikkilä and Kurunmäki 1987; Kivijärvi 1987; Laatikainen and Tikkanen 1987; Luukkainen 1985; Lähteenmäki 1987a; Lähteenmäki 1987b; Saarikoski 1987; Siegberg and Nilsson 1987; Toivonen 1982).

These are all descriptions of Norplant and reviews of previous studies. They also often include the author's experience and opinions. Three articles also present results of empirical studies on Norplant published in more detail elsewhere. The following is a summary of the recommendations in these articles which refer specifically to the use of Norplant in Finland.

General recommendations – restricted use in Finland

The authors generally do not believe that Norplant should replace any previous contraceptive method (Holma 1984; Holma 1987; Toivonen 1982; Toivonen 1985). The use in Finland is expected to be restricted and the main market area to be in the Third World (Holma 1984; Toivonen 1985; Erkkola 1983).

Norplant is described as effective, safe, long-acting, reversible, and not requiring constant motivation. (Toivonen 1985; Holma 1987). Holma (1987) describes Norplant as the most effective contraceptive method on the market.

Selection of potential users

Potential users of Norplant in Finland include, in principle, all women who need contraception, but especially women who have completed their families (Toivonen 1982; Holma 1987) and women who cannot use other methods (Holma 1987). Young women are thought to be less tolerant of bleeding irregularities and so several articles do not recommend Norplant as a first choice for them (Toivonen 1985; Holma 1987; Siegberg and Nilsson 1987). However, several authors mention that young women who do not use oral contraceptives successfully due to an irregular life style or negligence could be a target group for Norplant (Lähteenmäki 1987a; Siegberg and Nilsson 1987). The recommendation for older women is not clear. One author states that not enough is known to apply an upper age limit, but mentions that in his own practice he will not insert Norplant in women over 40 (Toivonen 1985). Another believes that older women might benefit from the extra progestin in Norplant (Holma 1987). Norplant is also recommended for contraception after abortion. It is not recommended for use after delivery because of the lack of information about the long-term effects on breast-fed infants (Heikkilä and Kurunmäki 1987). One author warns against the lowered effectiveness of Norplant if women use medication for epilepsy or rifampicin as treatment for tuberculosis (Haukkamaa M. 1987).

Attitudes towards side-effects, insertion and removal

Bleeding irregularities are described as rather frequent. It is believed, however, that good counselling and careful selection of users could help to overcome this problem (Toivonen 1982; Toivonen 1985).

Acceptance is reported to be good and continuation rates high in Finland (Holma, 1984; Holma 1987). Insertions are considered easy, but the need for correct insertion is stressed (Holma 1984; Toivonen 1985; Holma 1987). Removals are not believed to cause any problems (Holma 1984; Holma 1987), but the procedure is described in detail by one author (Holma 1987).

Discussion

Norplant in Finland: Norplant is of marginal importance in birth control in Finland. It is not possible to estimate the extent of use in the country from our survey. However, it is estimated that around 1% of women of fertile age use Norplant (Järvelä, Leiras Pharmaceuticals, personal communication 1989; Makkonen and Hemminki 1990). According to our survey, family planning clinics had higher expectations of Norplant at an early stage of use. The use seems to currently be stabilising at a lower level.

In this small sample of public family planning clinics, many of the public health centres surveyed did not provide Norplant six years after its introduction. This was particularly true for clinics in the Northern provinces.

In Finland, Norplant is considered a good method for carefully selected women. Its use is preceded by eliminating other forms of contraception and careful counselling about the possible side-effects and the surgical nature of insertion and removal procedures.

In comparison to the people interviewed in our survey, authors in Finnish medical journals seem to be rather optimistic about tolerance of side-effects and the ease of insertions and removals. Further research on side-effects, discontinuations and method failures in Finland would be needed to confirm our results.

There are clear indications that women have been more eager to try Norplant than physicians have been to prescribe it. Physicians believe that women's magazines give too positive a picture of the method. Women's curiosity about Norplant has also been confirmed in another Finnish survey in which women were asked which contraceptive method they would like to know more about. While only 1% used Norplant, 20% wanted to know more about it (Makkonen, personal communication 1991). We plan to look more closely at the information in women's magazines to see how the method is being portrayed.

Many practitioners seem rather frustrated with the situation. Women request Norplant and have high expectations of the method. Once the implants are inserted, women keep coming back because of side-effects such as irregular bleeding. The practitioners then need to counsel the woman to decide whether to try to live with the side-effects, treat them with more hormones, or to remove the implants. They say that this is often time consuming and difficult because of the woman's or their own ambivalence. Practitioners try to treat irregular bleeding with oral hormones, often with little success. Furthermore, removals are often time consuming and considered difficult. Our study does not allow us to interpret the attitudes of women towards Norplant. The fact that physicians have reservations does not necessarily mean that women share these negative attitudes. We plan to study women's experiences with Norplant in Finland in the near future.

We do not know of any studies of the safety of the treatment of bleeding irregularities caused by Norplant with oral hormones. Relatively higher concentrations of levonorgestrel are released during the early period of Norplant use. The addition of oral hormones may lead to a high dose of synthetic hormones. In Finland, these treatments are not included in any official protocol and physicians seem to resort to them fairly infrequently. The bleeding disturbances associated with Norplant use are, however, very common. A serious effort should be made to prevent the further spread of these treatments until their safety has been adequately assessed.

"Asocial women" were mentioned among the specific user groups. This group was also included in a commercial list of possible users given out by the manufacturer. In the United States, there is public discussion about this use (Goodman 1991a; Goodman 1991b; Purvis 1990; Anonymous 1991). In Finland, this discussion has not occurred. However, the role of the physician as a moral gatekeeper (Stevenson 1991) could also be questioned in Finland.

Norplant in Third World countries: Norplant has been considered a good contraceptive for Third World countries because "it is highly effective, safe, long-acting, convenient and easily motivated for women's use" (Holma 1984). However, the experience in Finland sheds some doubts on these assertions.

The Finnish experience of Norplant shows clearly that careful selection and counselling of women are required.

Norplant has been offered as a method of first choice on some occasions in Third World countries – if any choice was offered at all (Anonymous 1988; UBINIG 1990; Ward et al. 1990). The use is limited in Finland to very restricted groups of women, and users are selected very carefully. It does not replace any of the existing methods of contraception. The authorisation for use on the domestic Finnish market has, however, been important in the rapid expansion of Norplant's use in the Third World. It has enabled the manufacturer to use the WHO certification scheme for exports to Third World countries. Use in Finland also gives a "modern and Western" status to Norplant (UBINIG 1990; Morsy in this publication), which further facilitates its implementation in the Third World.

The method has proven to be reasonably safe in Finland. However, good access to continued medical care and removal on demand are needed because of the frequent side-effects. In our survey in Finland there were several reports of incorrect insertions and considerable difficulties with removals. In Third World countries Norplant has been provided in areas where few possibilities for return visits exist and where removal on demand does not always occur (Anonymous 1988; Garcia and Dacach 1992; Ministry of Public Health of Thailand 1988; Ward et al. 1990).

Norplant does not hinder the transmission of sexually transmitted diseases. The surgical procedures for insertion and removal may increase transmission of Hepatitis B and HIV infections if adequate hygienic standards cannot be met. These standards have not always been met (Ward et al. 1990). Medical safety – and eventually effectiveness, if the implant is not removed in time – may be lower in the conditions encountered in Third World countries.

Norplant is convenient to the extent that the method does not require daily user intake or frequent prescriptions by health professionals. However, bleeding irregularities are disturbing to Finnish women, and might be even more disturbing to women with less access to good health care.

Norplant is a long-acting contraceptive. In Finland this long-term character was considered a limiting factor in Norplant's use. Five years is a long time to space children. One may also question whether it is always an advantage in Third World countries. If so, is it an advantage for the women?

Norplant is a highly provider-dependent method both at the beginning of its use and at its end. The fact that even in Finland asocial women were seen as a special target group for Norplant alerts us to possible abuse in more repressive societies. As Purvis (1990) asks, "Are the women deemed unfit for motherhood" deemed fit for Norplant use?

Box 1

Pharmaca Fennica 1989 Entry
(translated from the Finnish)

Norplant 6 x 36 mg implants
Levonorgestrel 6 x 36 mg, Consist. q.s.

Levonorgestrel is a progestin that has been used for a long time for contraception in "mini-pills" and in combined oral contraceptives. When administered alone, at a dose of 30 mcg/day, levonorgestrel thickens the cervical mucus and inhibits sperm penetration into the uterus; inhibits ovulation in over half of the menstrual cycles; and suppresses the endometrium, thereby inhibiting the implantation of the ovum. Together these mechanisms protect effectively against pregnancy. Contraception with progestins only is especially advisable when the administration of oestrogens is not desirable. Implants are an advisable form of administration when aiming at long-term contraception.

Norplant 6 x 36 mg consists of six rods inserted subdermally in a woman's upper arm. The implants are covered by a silicone widely used in medicine through which levonorgestrel is released slowly: initially at a rate of 70 mcg/day, with the amount stabilising after the first year to 30 mcg/day. The implants are effective for five years. These results are from a multinational trial carried out in Finland, Denmark, the USA, Brazil, Thailand and Egypt.

In a large five-year-long multi-centre trial with a total of 2,380 woman years (992 users) the pregnancy rate for the first year was 0.3 and the cumulative rate for five years was 2.7/100 woman years. The following yearly rates are from a recent analysis:

year	user-years	pregnancy rate
1	1455	0.3
2	982	0.6
3	642	1.4
4	414	1.2
5	282	0

The discontinuation rate because of irregular bleeding during the first year of use has been 6-12% in different trials.
Bleeding irregularities have not been shown to cause any danger to health, since quantitative blood loss or decline in haemoglobin values have not been shown. The most common disturbance encountered has been irregular bleeding. Disturbances diminish markedly after the first three months of use. After the first year of use the continuation rates have been 77-90%. Fertility returned to normal when the rods were removed.

Indications: Contraception
Dosage: Six implants are inserted subdermally in the inside of the upper arm.

Period of administration: The implants are inserted during menstrual bleeding, at the latest within seven days from the start of bleeding, when the possibility of pregnancy is low.

Use during pregnancy and lactation: If the patient becomes pregnant during the use of Norplant, the implants must be removed immediately. Results from animal trials have shown that high concentrations of gestagens may cause masculinisation of female foetuses. These findings do not, however, necessarily apply to human beings, especially not for the low concentrations with Norplant use.
The use of Norplant during lactation has been studied in a limited number of patients. Small amounts of levonorgestrel are released into the milk. Although clear harmful effects on the health of the infants have not been observed, the use of Norplant implants is not desirable during lactation.

Contraindications: Breast cancer, other hormone-dependent cancers, unexplained uterine bleeding, previous thromboembolic disease, active liver disease.

Side-effects: Side-effects typical for progestins may occur: irregularities of the menstrual cycle (frequent, irregular, long-lasting, abundant or scarce bleeding, spotting, amenorrhoea); headaches, also migraine; dizziness; nervousness; depression; changes in libido; loss of appetite; nausea; acne; and weight gain.

Interactions: The effectiveness of Norplant implants may be reduced in women using drugs that induce steroid metabolism, for example: barbiturates, phenytoin, carbamazepin, rifampicin.

Observation: Before inserting the implants, a gynaecological examination including breast examination and exclusion of pregnancy must be performed. Control visits should take place three months after insertion, and thereafter once a year. If no menstrual bleeding has occurred within six weeks from the beginning of the previous bleeding episode, the possibility of pregnancy must be excluded. Liver function tests may need to be performed in women with a history of disturbances in liver function. The glucose tolerance may change, and therefore the glucose balance of diabetic patients should be monitored. If lower abdominal pain occurs in connection with irregular bleeding (especially if a menstrual period is missed after a long period of irregular bleeding) the possibility of an ectopic pregnancy should be taken into consideration. The risk for ectopic pregnancy is higher in patients with a history of ectopic pregnancy. The implants must be removed if the woman gets migraine-type headaches for the first time, exceptionally strong headache, disturbances in vision (shivering vision), icterus or increased blood pressure. Norplant implants are not recommended for women with recent disturbances in the menstrual cycle (such as oligomenorrhoea or amenorrhoea), women with seborrhoea, acne, problems with weight, polycystic ovaries, or high levels of cholesterol, nor for women who smoke and are over 40. The effectiveness of Norplant is markedly lower in women who weigh more than 70 kilograms.

Period of use: Five years. After five years the implants must be removed. If the woman wants to continue using the method, a new set of implants may be inserted immediately.

Storage: At room temperature, protected from moisture, the shelf life is five years.

Packing: 6 x 36 mg (soft, white rod, Norplant 6 x 36 mg rod is 34 mm long, 10 mm shorter than Norplant 2 x 70 mg rod).

Appendix 1 Interview Questions

Questions for providers:

1. How many years have you worked in family planning?
   How many sets of Norplant have you inserted? (Specify between the two types of Norplant)
   How many have you removed? (Specify Norplant types)

2. Have you received practical teaching in insertions/removals?
   If so, who organised these teaching sessions?
   From which information sources have you learned about Norplant?
   From which sources do women learn about Norplant?

3. How do you select the women to whom you recommend Norplant for contraception?
   To which women do you recommend Norplant?
   Do you recommend Norplant as a method of first choice?
   To whom do you not recommend Norplant?
   Have you inserted Norplant for women you consider to be "asocial"?
   What kind of information on Norplant do you give to potential users?

4. What side-effects have you encountered in your own practice during Norplant use?
   What is the frequency of irregular bleeding?
   Have you prescribed any drugs to treat irregular bleeding?
   If yes, what kind and for how long?
   What is the frequency of amenorrhoea?
   Have you prescribed any drugs to treat amenorrhoea?
   If yes, what kind and for how long?
   In case of amenorrhoea, do you perform a pregnancy test?

5. List the reasons for discontinuation in your own practice.
   (e.g., irregular bleeding, amenorrhoea, other side-effects, ovarian cysts, wish to get pregnant).
   Have ovarian cysts been a reason for discontinuation?

6. Have you encountered pregnancies during Norplant use? Number?
   Did they continue? Were there any ectopic pregnancies?

7. Insertions and removals:
   What is the average time required for the procedures?
   Any infections encountered at the site? Damage to rods?
   Have several sessions ever been needed for removal? Other difficulties?
   What is your general opinion of the procedures?

8. Are you satisfied with the method?
   What is your impression about the women's satisfaction with the method?
   Do you think the method is becoming more popular in Finland?

Questions for non-providers:

1. How many years have you worked in family planning?
   How many sets of Norplant have you inserted? (Specify between the two types of Norplant)
   How many have you removed? (Specify Norplant types)
   Do you have any personal experience in your practice with patients who use Norplant (e.g., control visits)?
   What do you know from others' experience?

2. Why don't you insert Norplant in your family planning practice?
   Are you familiar with the method?
   Have you had training to provide the method?
   Have you attended any presentations on Norplant by drug representatives?

3. What do you think of Norplant?
   What is your impression of the method?
   Is there something you don't like about the method?

4. Do you think you would be interested in providing Norplant in the future?
   How do you see Norplant's place among the other contraceptives available in Finland?
   Do you see women who request the method?
   If so, do you refer them to somewhere else for Norplant?

References

Anonymous. "Hilltribe Women Welcome New Birth Control Method." *Bangkok Post*, 18 October 1988.

Anonymous. "Plan to Induce Welfare Moms to Use Implant." *San Francisco Chronicle*, 9 February 1991:7.

Erkkola, R. "Naisen iän ja synnyttäneisyyden vaikutus ehkäisymenetelmän valintaan." *Suomen lääkärilehti* 1983; (38):1993-1998.

Garcia G. and Dacach S. "Norplant – 5 Years Later." *A Question of Control: Women's perspectives on the development and use of contraceptive technologies.* Mintzes B.(ed), WEMOS/HAI, 1992.

Goodman E. "Norplant: Incentive or Coercion?" *San Francisco Chronicle*, 19 February 1991a:15.

Goodman E. "Help to Plan Family, Not Control the Women." *Herald Tribune*, 20 February 1991b:9.

Haddad W., Lewin B., Vienonen M. "Position paper on Family Planning." Copenhagen: WHO Regional Office for Europe, 1984.

Haukkamaa M. "Hormonaalinen ehkäisy ja muu lääkehoito." *Duodecim* 1987; (103): 598-602.

Heikkilä M., Kurunmäki H. "Raskaudenkeskeytyksen ja synnytyksen jälkeinen ehkäisy." *Duodecim* 1987; (103): 588-591.

Holma P. "Ihonalaiset ehkäisykapselit." *Suomen lääkärilehti* 1984; (39): 406-411.

Holma P. "Ihonalaiset hormonikapselit." *Duodecim* 1987; (103):538-545.

Kivijärvi A. "Ehkäisymenetelmien seuranta käytännössä." *Duodecim* 1987; (103): 609-614.

Laatikainen T., Tikkanen MJ. "Ehkäisypillereiden metaboliset vaikutukset." *Duodecim* 1987; (103): 532-537.

Lähteenmäki P. "Ehkäisymenetelmän valinta." *Duodecim* 1987; (103): 513-515.

Lähteenmäki P. "Hormonaalisen ehkäisyn hyödyt ja riskit." *Duodecim* 1987; (103): 525-531.

Lääketietokeskus: 1990 Lääkevalmisteet. Helsinki: Pharmaca Fennica, 1989.

Luukkainen T. "Perhesuunnittelu." *Duodecim* 1985; (101): 1428-1430.

Makkonen K., Hemminki E. "Different Contraceptive Practices: Use of Contraceptives in Finland and Other Nordic Countries in the 1970s and 1980s." *Scandinavian Journal of Social Medicine* 1991; (19):32-38.

Ministry of Public Health in Thailand. "Norplant Acceptability in Thailand. Report on a Survey of Acceptors in Clinical Trials." Unpublished. Ministry of Public Health, Research and Evaluation Unit, Family Health Division, Department of Health. June 1988.

Purvis A. "A pill that gets under the skin. Norplant could spur birth control – and stir controversy. *Time*, 24 December 1990:45.

Saarikoski S. "Krooniset sairaudet ja ehkäisy." *Duodecim* 1987; (103): 593-597.

Siegberg R., Nilsson C.G. "Teini-iäisten raskauden ehkäisy." *Duodecim* 1987; (103): 584-587.

Stephenson S.T, Clair P., Wagner M.G. "Turkey-baster Babies: A View from Europe." *Milbank Quarterly* 1991; (69): 45-50.

Toivonen Juhani. "Hormonaalisen kontraseption tulevaisuuden menetelmät." *Suomen lääkärilehti* 1982; (37):2495-2496.

Toivonen Juhani. "Ihonalainen ehkäisykapseli." *Duodecim* 1985; (101): 1336-1338.

UBINIG. "Research report. Norplant, the Five Year Needle: An Investigation of the Norplant Trial in Bangladesh from the User's Perspective." *Issues in Reproductive and Genetic Engineering* 1990; (3):211-228.

Vienonen M. "Ehkäisyn käyttö Suomessa." *Duodecim* 1987 (103): 515-517.

Ward J.S., Poernomo Sigit Sidi I, Simmons R., Simmons G.B. "Service Delivery Systems and Quality of Care in the Implementation of Norplant in Indonesia." Unpublished report. New York: The Population Council, 1990.

Norplant – five years later[1] [Brazil]

by Giselle Garcia and Solange Dacach

The research project, "Norplant – five years later", was carried out by the Network for the Defense of the Human Species (REDEH) to assess the condition of Brazilian women who were the subjects of pre-introductory trials involving the long-acting hormonal contraceptive Norplant.

Norplant was first tested on Brazilian women in 1975, when it was introduced by Professor Elsimar Coutinho of the University of Bahia. He began the tests without consultation or authorisation from the Ministry of Health, although this is a legal requirement for experiments involving human beings.

In 1984 Professor Aníbal Faúndes of the University of Campinas (UNICAMP) obtained permission to carry out a pre-introductory trial of Norplant on 2,000 women.

As a result of irregularities in the trials and protests from the women's movement, the Ministry of Health prohibited further trials of Norplant in January 1986 (Ministry of Health 1986). At that time, tests involving approximately 3,500 women were being carried out by family planning clinics in various states. Many of these clinics were situated in teaching hospitals.

The Ministry of Health concluded that the research did not follow basic international norms of ethics and safety required for human clinical trials of new products. In addition, a commission was set up to assist women who had taken part or were still taking part in the trials.

It is clear that the government authorities did not carry out the recommendations of the Ministry of Health, as stated in the report of the working commission appointed to look into research on Norplant. The

---

1 This article is an updated and expanded version of "Norplant – 5 Years later" by G. Garcia and S. Dacach, published in: *A Question of Control: Women's perspectives on the development and use of contraceptive technologies.* Mintzes B. (ed), WEMOS/HAI 1992.

commission's recommendations included the following (Ministry of Health 1987):

- Development of criteria for supervision of the Norplant research teams and clinical-gynaecological assessment of women involved in the research;
- Removal of implants from women with clinical histories demonstrating incompatibility;
- Developing strategies to assist women using the method;
- Developing strategies to guarantee free access to alternative contraceptives and information on alternatives in all centres participating in Norplant research;
- Public reporting of the commission's findings, to reach Norplant users and the population as a whole.

Follow-up study of women involved in trials in Rio de Janeiro

In Rio de Janeiro UNICAMP authorised two private family planning organisations to carry out trials of Norplant involving 309 women: 253 took part in the trial through the Research Centre for Integrated Assistance to Women and Children (CPAIMC) and 56 through the Civil Society for Family Well-being in Brazil (BEMFAM). All of these women had Norplant implanted between July 1984 and January 1986.

In July 1990, REDEH began a follow-up study of women who received implants during the trials. Aware of the incidence of alterations in the menstrual cycle during Norplant use, we were especially concerned with assessing the physical and psychological impact of these changes on sexuality, marital relationships and daily life. We also wanted to explore the meaning of menstruation to these women.

We had lists of names and addresses of women who had taken part in the trials. We wrote to 309 women in the Rio de Janeiro area. The post returned 50 letters because women had moved and had left no forwarding address. Many of the women who took part in trials live in slums. The researchers did not take into consideration the frequent migration of slum inhabitants when enrolling them in trials requiring long-term follow-up.

After two months, we initiated a search for the remaining women. We were only able to contact 52 of the 309 women who took part in trials in the Rio de Janeiro area. We interviewed 22 women in our clinic and 30 in home visits.

We contacted the women six and a half years after the introductory trial had begun. Sixteen of the 52 women we contacted still had Norplant in their arm. Fourteen of these women had the implants for more than five years, although the implant should be removed after five years. The time period ranged from just over five years to five years and eleven months. The remaining two women had the implants for almost five years (four years, nine months and four years, ten months).[2] Some women did not know who to turn to for removal because the doctors originally involved in the research had left and other doctors did not know how to remove the implants.

The discovery that these women had been abandoned by the researchers undertaking Norplant trials was the most immediate and serious result of our study. There was a clear need for immediate action. These women have received no assistance whatsoever from those responsible for the research on Norplant.

We could not interview the women and leave them with Norplant still implanted. REDEH arranged for doctors to be trained so that the women who still had Norplant past its expiry date could have the implants removed. However, an important question is who will foot the bill.

We were only able to contact a small proportion of the women who had taken part in trials. What happened to the other women? Who will contact them and pay for removal of Norplant from those women who still have the implants? What has happened to the women in other parts of Brazil who also took part in Norplant trials?

Interview results

The reasons women gave for using Norplant

Many reasons were given for using Norplant, showing the lack of alternatives for women who seek to avoid having children "at any price". The official doctrine of demographic control blames women who have many children for the social and economic misery of Brazil. There are no policies to guarantee the population's basic necessities for health, education, nourishment and housing.

Many of the women who took part in the studies of Norplant live in conditions of extreme poverty in the Favelas (shanty towns) of Caju, Jacarezinho and Catumbi and the suburbs of Vila Sao Luiz and Duque de Caxias. These areas are subject to continuous conflict between the police and drug dealers, another motive for women to avoid having more children.

---

2 This is a correction of the information reported on this study in *A Question of Control* (Garcia and Dacach 1992), which states that fifteen women still had Norplant when interviewed and does not differentiate between the women who had the implants less than five years or more than five years.

In at least one case, the clinic strongly promoted the use of Norplant to a woman who ended up taking part in the trial:

> "I didn't go to BEMFAM for Norplant. I went for a preventive. But I was sent to a girl who said she was a nurse. Then she started talking about Norplant. Nowadays I know what "inducing" means. They induce people. That day I met various girls, young girls who had never had children and were using Norplant."

Selection of trial participants
Among the women we interviewed there were: women who had never been pregnant before using Norplant; women with severe mental disorders, including visual hallucinations and a history of psychiatric hospitalisation; alcoholics; women with hypertension; smokers; malnourished women and a diabetic who was undiagnosed at the time. These women should not have been included in a clinical trial according to medical or ethical criteria. This is a small subset of women involved in the Norplant trials and gives no overall idea of how many women were included who should not have participated in a trial.

Experiences of being abandoned by doctors and researchers
The women who still had the implant when we interviewed them suffered anxiety because of the absence of the doctors responsible for the trials. Many of these women were confused and unsure of their fate with the implants still in place after the five year period of effectiveness. They did not know what contraceptive to use or had gone back to the pill although they had side-effects from the pill in the past. Their insecurity and sense of abandonment were evident:

> "I don't know where they are (the doctors)...I'm longing to find them."

> "...We got there, me and my friend, and didn't see the doctor. He wasn't there any more. The girl couldn't even tell us where he is. So we started thinking: well, why isn't the doctor there?"

> "...I'm worried. I even cried at work this week because they told me a woman had died from Norplant."

"...I would like to take it out...because the doctor said you shouldn't keep it after five years and so I don't know if it works or not."

Many side-effects were reported

Of the 52 women interviewed, 45 reported experiencing side-effects from Norplant. These included: changes in the menstrual cycle, acne, headaches, temporary visual disturbances, ovarian cysts, breast lumps, weight changes, increased blood pressure, increase in body hair, hair loss, insomnia, anxiety, and loss of sexual desire.

Menstrual changes

Menstrual cycle changes were the most common side-effect and were experienced by 36 women, with or without additional problems.

The primary reason the women used a contraceptive was to avoid pregnancy. Lack of menstruation or increases in the intervals between menstrual cycles were sometimes alarming because of the possibility of pregnancy. However, if the women were told by a doctor that this was a result of Norplant, they considered it normal.

An increase in menstrual flow or a shortened interval between cycles caused profound displeasure because, "it's bad to have sex when you're menstruating," "my husband doesn't like it", "it's disgusting".

Here are excerpts of women's descriptions of menstrual problems:

"It came several times a month and for a long time. I menstruated much more than usual."

"I didn't menstruate much before and it got much less. There were months when it didn't come at all...It didn't come for three or four months. Then it came, but just a dirty mark, just a trace, but every month I had pains, signs of it coming. After five years it started coming twice a month."

"There were months that I menstruated for 20 days."

"It comes and I don't know when it'll stop. It comes a lot, really heavy and completely uncontrolled...These five years...once I menstruated for almost a whole month."

"I had no way of stopping it. My sister-in-law ran to her house and got the tablecloth and stuffed it between my legs. I was green

> already, I couldn't take any more. He [a person mentioned earlier in the interview] put me in the car and took me to the hospital. I had to stay eight days on a drip. Four different people here from Jacare donated blood to me."

Effect on sexual relationships and libido

Norplant interfered in the daily lives of these women in various ways. Some experienced excessive menstruation which interfered with their sexual relationships. Others experienced a decrease in libido:

> "I felt less desire. When you're menstruating twice a month you get sluggish."

> "There's one thing...most of all...I just lost all my feelings...I didn't feel aroused by anything, didn't feel that urge. I hardly felt any pleasure at all."

> "After Norplant I didn't feel anything. I became frigid. Before Norplant I was a real woman. After I put it in I stopped being a woman. All I'm good for is working and feeding the kids."

Inadequate medical follow-up

Many women did not have follow-up medical exams following insertion of Norplant. The low rate of attendance of health services for gynaecological and clinical follow-up among the women interviewed is related to many factors:

- carelessness with one's own health;
- priority given to work and children;
- lack of money to attend health services;
- use of health services near home;
- they did not know the new addresses of the family planning services (BEMFAM and CPAIMC), which moved without further notice;
- lack of awareness of the need for periodic check-ups because they were inadequately informed by health workers during Norplant insertion;
- other health personnel in private or public institutions refused to provide care because they were unfamiliar with Norplant;
- those women who had Norplant removed no longer associated continuing health problems with Norplant use.

Individual situations

These are the stories of three of the women we interviewed. Two of these women clearly should have had Norplant removed when they first requested it. The third woman was able to have the implants removed after lying and saying she wished to become pregnant. Their stories are included because they describe situations which should never have happened.

One of the women interviewed was 28 years old and epileptic and had been taking medicines for epilepsy since age 14. She had previously become pregnant with an IUD in place and had miscarried when the IUD was removed. She was already a patient at CPAIMC before having Norplant inserted. After using Norplant for four months, during which time she experienced menstrual cycle disturbances, decrease in libido, red spots on her legs and many epileptic crises, she developed amenorrhoea and suspected pregnancy. She went to CPAIMC where a doctor told her she couldn't possibly be pregnant. After having a positive pregnancy test, she returned to the clinic and was given the same answer: "This is impossible, You must have developed a myoma." Eventually, in the fourth month of pregnancy, the doctor detected her pregnancy and removed the implants.

Another woman, also 28 years old, who lived in a slum, Jacarezinho, had used Norplant for nine months. She also received the implants from CPAIMC. Since having Norplant inserted, she had menstruated constantly for nine months and said that she had lost 22 kilos. She returned to CPAIMC several times to have the implants removed and was systematically refused. She described her situation in a television programme, threatening the institution with a scandal, and was eventually able to have the capsules removed. When we interviewed her, the state of her health was shocking. The many health problems she reported prevented her from being able to work. As a result of her inability to work, she was very poor and had difficulty supporting and feeding herself and her three children.

She was taken to the Fernando Magalhaes Municipal Institute for Women, assessed and given medical assistance to treat persistent haemorrhageing and psychological support and therapy for emotional instability. She eventually needed to have a hysterectomy.

A third woman, 38 years old and living at Baixada Fluminense, had obtained Norplant from BEMFAM and used it for 18 months. She had the implants removed after developing amenorrhoea and migraines. To convince the doctor to remove the capsules, she lied and said she had decided to get pregnant. Since the removal, she has never had a normal menstrual cycle. She began to try to get pregnant without success and started infertility treatment. She was diagnosed as having a precocious menopause. She was previously fertile and has a son. She has since initiated a lawsuit claiming that her sterility was caused by Norplant. It is not possible to prove that Norplant has made her sterile; however, we do not dismiss this possibility.

Comments

What is a "normal" side-effect?

We perceived two important aspects which go together when a woman accepts a new contraceptive method: 1) the desire not to have children is strong enough to warrant taking a risk or various risks; 2) a woman's ignorance of her own body allows her to interpret changes according to imposed criteria and changing concepts of normality. We would like to emphasise the distortion of the idea of normality. For every complaint, women received the same answer from the doctor: "This is quite normal."

> "There were months when I menstruated for 20 days. So he (the doctor) said 'it will get to be less over time'...and I saw that it really did go down to 12 days...It wasn't really a haemorrhage. He said: 'It's normal. Keep calm and be patient.' Nearly five years went by like that."

> "I thought it was normal [menstruation lasting 15 days after the 3rd month of Norplant use]...I thought it was normal because I didn't feel strange...The blood was normal...It didn't come in bits."

The way in which women perceived changes in their cycle and other side-effects as normal was further confirmed in that most of the women accepted full responsibility themselves, sparing the researchers of any blame:

> "They told me I might get much thinner or fatter, have headaches, feel sick. If I suffer from headaches, that's my problem, not the doctor's. I have to accept it. It was me that wanted it. The doctor didn't force me to put it in...Wasn't it me who decided to have it? It's our own problem."

> "I knew it was an experiment with risks, not too big. They said it was just sickness, giddiness, cloudy vision."

> "I put in this thing in full consciousness. The paper I signed said there would be menstrual problems for a while. And a lady doctor said to me: 'Look, this will get better over time.' It's like when you go to the doctor thinking you have a serious illness and he says to you: 'This isn't anything serious. It'll get better.' You know, you convince yourself you'll get better, so the only way is to keep going or you'll get desperate. That's what happened."

Norplant and women's sense of time
The researcher's lack of respect for the body and physiology are apparent in the dismissive attitude towards the complete time change in the menstrual cycle caused by Norplant. This is also apparent in the attitudes of many of the women who took part in the trials towards the changes in their menstrual cycles: three days, fifteen days a month, once every three or six months, twice a month; all are considered normal.

Although universal, the concept of time is a cultural construct. Each society experiences time in a particular way. It's up to the individual to adapt, submit or to refuse this time scale. Frequently, social time interferes with or imposes limits on biological time and ecological time.

We are going through a period in which some people consider birth control to be the solution for humanity's problems. This aim is imposed at the expense of women's right to experience their own physiological cycle. Women have a natural biological time governed by the menstrual cycle. This is essential to their health.

Final considerations: time for action

REDEH, together with the women's movement and official health institutions, led a series of actions to bring public attention to the abandonment of women involved in the Norplant trials and to call for adequate medical attention for these women. The following institutions collaborated with our proposal to assist these women:

- Fernando Magalhaes Municipal Institute for Women (FMMIW)
- The State Council for Women's Rights – CEDIM
- The Regional Medical Council of Rio de Janeiro
- The Regional Pharmaceutical Council of Rio de Janeiro
- The General Hospital of Jacarepagua

Just 22 of the women interviewed went to FMMIW for medical care: nine with Norplant, which was removed, and 13 without it. We do not know what has happened to the seven women who still had Norplant when we interviewed them and did not go to FMMIW.

The extracted capsules were sent to the National Institute of Health Control, a Ministry of Health organisation, in order to evaluate the quality and quantity of hormonal residues. Seventeen months after the initial request, no answer has been provided, in spite of persistent inquiries from REDEH and FMMIW.

The press coverage in December 1990 of Norplant's approval and commercialisation in the United States brought an immediate response from

REDEH. We contacted the press and the women's movement and sought to bring public attention to the information we obtained about the state of health of women who used Norplant in Rio de Janeiro. We hope this publicity will lead to similar actions through the various states of Brazil, where more than 3,500 women were the subjects of this catastrophic experiment.

Epilogue - *The Norplant Route*[3] and reproductive rights

In 1991, the high frequency of sterilisation of Brazilian women began to be discussed throughout the country. In Rio de Janeiro, a Parliamentary Committee was set up at the Legislative Assembly to investigate who was responsible for mass sterilisation. Solange Dacach coordinated the work of this investigative committee. The third woman described in the section on individual situations, who became sterile after Norplant use, was asked to testify to the committee. This started a debate on the invisibility of chemical sterilisation.

The Investigative Parliamentary Committee concluded that both BEMFAM and CPAIMC in Rio, as well as other health services, were responsible for performing abusive surgical sterilisation. The Rio de Janeiro Civil Police Secretary has ordered a police investigation at DEAM (Delegacia Especial de Atendimento a Mulher) after accepting the decision of the Investigative Parliamentary Committee. DEAM is a special police task force set up to assist women, which was created in response to pressure from the feminist movement.

DEAM has begun a police investigation and is asking women who have been involuntarily sterilised to testify. They are also accepting testimony from women who participated in the Norplant trials.

In Rio de Janeiro, the state of health and denial of rights of women who took part in the trials of Norplant points to a thread that deserves investigation – not just in the sociological sense – but also in the sense of a police investigation.

---

3 *The Norplant Route* is the title of a book soon to be published by the authors of this article, describing their research on Norplant and the "arrangements" legitimising the trials.

References

Ministry of Health, Brazil. National Division of Health Control over Drugs (DIMED). *A Long List of restrictions*, Ministry of Health, January 1986.

Ministry of Health, Brazil. *Report of the Working Commission for the Reassessment of the Norplant Research*, appointed by Ministerial Dispatch M/S. 32/86. Brasilia, 1987.

Inserting Norplant at all cost?

A case report of a Norplant training session in Thailand

by Judith Richter, Piengporn Panut-Ampon, and Prasert Kiatboonsri

The Population Council's Norplant introduction programme

"In the past the introduction of newly developed contraceptives to developing countries has been haphazard and incomplete, and has not given sufficient attention to a variety of political, economic, social, management and user satisfaction issues that need to be addressed at the international and national levels" – such were the concerns expressed by the Population Council in a background paper on the introduction of Norplant into family planning programmes (Population Council 1988). The paper continues "...the emergence of heightened sensitivity to contraceptives, and even organised opposition to certain contraceptive technologies, has made the need for careful, well-articulated introduction efforts essential".

How, specifically, did the Population Council intend to dispel the fears of women that the provision of the new long-acting, provider-dependent implants might turn out to be to their detriment?

The report refers to a comprehensive Norplant introduction programme set up by the Council since 1983 in collaboration with a number of other agencies. It mentions "over 700 Thai physicians [who] were trained in insertion and removal techniques" (Population Council 1998, p. 7) as a visible symbol of the success of this scheme.

However, our findings from an informal survey in a Thai district hospital cast serious doubts on the Population Council's ability to guarantee the quality of the training sessions at hospitals and clinics where services will be provided.

Training in a Thai district hospital

In June 1989 a health professional from a Thai district hospital contacted our public health research and information centre, the Drug Information for Action Centre in Bangkok. He had read our articles on Norplant and was aware of unresolved issues concerning Norplant's use and the risks of overenthusiastic promotion of the method. He told us that his hospital had participated in the government's training programme for Norplant provision a year and a half beforehand. Many of the women participating had already requested the removal of the capsules. This led him to wonder about their satisfaction with the method. He invited us to make an evaluation of the training programme in his hospital.

The training session was held in December 1986 in a modern district hospital in central Thailand. A physician from the area had participated in a Ministry of Public Health training session in Bangkok to learn to train other physicians. On his return, he provided Norplant training to physicians in the district hospital. During one month, 101 women received Norplant free of charge. Most insertions were done during one day in late December when over sixty women were brought to the hospital on specially hired pick-up trucks. A nurse later recalled that the women behaved as if they were coming to "a big party".

Research methodology

We had planned to assess the satisfaction of the women with Norplant by reviewing their medical records and by interviewing a representative sample of women. However, we soon realised that it would be impossible to obtain any statistically significant results. Many records were missing; others were less than complete. Our intention to interview a representative sample of women was shattered when we were told that at least half of the women had been prostitutes from two well-known local brothels. There was little hope of tracing these women due to difficulties of access and the high migration rate of this social group.

We therefore decided to concentrate on the quality of service provided instead of trying to assess user satisfaction with the method. We decided to evaluate the women's medical records – however incomplete – and to complement the information by interviewing the nurse in charge of family planning. She had been present during the training sessions.

The interview and the review of medical records took place one and a half years after the training session. We used the following five questions to focus the interview and examination of medical records:

- To what extent was the women's choice voluntary and based on full information about Norplant *and* other contraceptive methods?
- What was the quality of:
  - the pre-insertions service?
  - the insertion procedure?
  - the follow-up service?
  - the removal service?

Information provided prior to insertion

Our first question to the nurse was what type of information the women were given before deciding to use Norplant and who had provided the information.

Most of the women had come following a promotional campaign by the District Public Health Office which emphasised the long-term efficacy of the method. The nurse believed that the main informational/promotional tools had been a video and posters. The adverse effects of the method were described as similar to those of hormonal injections, which are usually seen as unimportant in Thailand. A minority of the women had been recruited by the hospital through the distribution of leaflets in front of the hospital or through suggestions to women in the maternity ward to try out this "new method". The nurse could not recall any more detailed counselling received by the women before the insertion of the implants.

We wondered how informed and voluntary the choice of the women might have been, considering the disproportionately high number of prostitutes. Prostitution is officially illegal in Thailand. Had these women been instructed that Norplant was the method of choice for them? Had their illegal status been used to pressure them to come to the training session? The nurse could not answer these questions.

We could not evaluate the quality of the written material as none was available. The hospital had run out of leaflets a long time before. However, we found that other information leaflets provided to the public in Thailand were less than optimal. For example, bleeding disturbances are the only adverse effect mentioned in the information leaflet on Norplant distributed by the Planned Parenthood Association of Thailand at approximately the same time.

Pre-insertion service

To verify that Norplant is really the most appropriate method for a particular woman and to ensure its safe use, health workers need to ask about a woman's socio-demographic background: her age, number of children, desire for more children, etc. They must also take a thorough medical history and provide a medical check-up.

According to the manufacturer of Norplant, this should include a gynaecological and breast exam. The provider must also make sure that the woman is not pregnant (Leiras Pharmaceuticals n.d.).

The records revealed an alarming disregard for these precautions. In fact, the guidelines used during the training session did not include any gynaecological examination nor ruling out of pregnancy.

At the time of the training, the Thai Ministry of Public Health recommended Norplant mainly for women nearing the end of childbearing age. However, the records which were left at the centre showed that 17 women were younger than 18. One woman was 14, six were 15, six were 16 and four were 17 at the time of insertion. A number of records had been thrown away, so it is impossible to know how many women in total were under 18. However, these records indicate that at least 17% of the women were under 18. Moreover, despite guidelines which explicitly prohibit enrolment of women over 45 (Ministry of Public Health 1988), two women were 49 years old when they had Norplant inserted.

Many of the records did not contain any medical data. When we pointed this out to the nurse we interviewed, she answered that, "the nurse who was responsible for the medical check-up during the main training day just filled in the questionnaires. She did not do any examinations – at most she took the woman's blood pressure." She claimed that in many cases where the data had been filled in, no medical history may have been taken and no check-up provided. Even apparent contraindications did not deter the trainees from inserting the implant. Although the official guidelines explicitly prohibit the use of Norplant by women with a systolic blood pressure reading of over 140, one woman was recorded to have had a systolic blood pressure of 150.

Insertion service

This survey could not provide any information on the quality of the insertion service. One important unresolved question is whether there was sufficient time to sterilise the trocars (the thick needles used for Norplant insertion) during the training day involving more than 60 women.

Follow-up service

Two elements of follow-up are essential to ensure the continued safety of this long-acting hormonal contraceptive. First, women should be informed which symptoms of adverse effects indicate that they should return to discuss their situation with a health professional. They should also be encouraged to feel free to return for consultation if they experience any health problem which they fear may be due to the method. Secondly, they should be invited to come for periodical medical check-ups[1]. Leiras recommends return visits three months after the insertion and once a year afterwards.

The nurse told us that the women were instructed not to have intercourse for five to seven days after insertion and not to wash the insertion site until the wound was dry. They were also encouraged to return if they experienced any problem with the method. The medical records did not show any adverse drug reactions despite the nurse's assurances that many women had returned because of complaints or for early removal because of side-effects. No arrangements were made for regular medical check-up.

Removal service

Norplant users are completely dependent on health workers for removal. It is therefore essential that no obstacles be raised if the woman asks for early removal for any reason. It is also necessary to have an effective recall system to trace women five years after the insertion of the capsules and to remind them of the necessity of removal.

How easy was it for the women to have Norplant removed? The nurse believed that women who desired early removal encountered no particular obstacles. She believed that by the time of the interview, a year and a half after the training session, most of the women had already requested the removal of the implants. However, it was impossible for us to make even a rough estimate of the percentage of women having undergone the removal procedure. Not a single case of early removal had been recorded. The nurse explained that in some cases of early removal the records had been removed and thrown away and in other cases not. This made it impossible even to infer the number of removals by subtracting the remaining records from the initial 101 Norplant users.

---

1 For details of the instruction necessitating a return visit, see Leiras Pharmaceuticals *Norplant Contraceptive Implants*, p. 22.

As already mentioned, no reasons for early removal were recorded. The nurse said that most of the women had cited problems with prolonged bleeding or spotting. The nurse commented that although spotting is a relatively minor adverse effect, it was the main reason for removal because nearly half of the women selected for the training were prostitutes and could not afford to lose working days because of spotting. She told us that most of the prostitutes had kept the capsules only for a few months before returning to the hospital and insisting strongly on early removal.

Other reasons for removal included dizziness, headache, numbness of the arm, or the desire to have a child. The nurse wondered whether the women who had justified their request for early removal with the desire to have a child had, in fact, wanted to avoid discussing their real reasons.

The nurse had kept personal notes regarding technical difficulties with removal. They indicated that in at least two cases the physicians had not been able to remove all six capsules. In one case, two capsules remained in the woman's arm, in the other case three. The nurse believed that these difficulties had occurred because the insertion was too deep. In one of these cases, the physician had to stop because of heavy bleeding. He told the woman not to worry about the two remaining capsules as the remaining hormone level would not interfere with her capacity to conceive.

It is important to carefully follow up Norplant users so they can be contacted when the implants are no longer effective. How concerned were the providers about the need to set up an effective mechanism to trace the Norplant users and remind them of the need to return for removal five years after the insertion? We could not find any evidence of such a mechanism in this hospital.

We would like to emphasise that the training session in this hospital covered insertion only and did not include training for removal. The physicians were left to manage as best as they could as the cases presented themselves after the training period. By June 1988, none of the trained physicians remained at the hospital. In most cases a male nurse was performing the Norplant removals.

The provision for removal within this training was far from ideal. We are concerned that efforts to establish appropriate removal services may decline when Norplant provision takes place within the routine family planning setting, rather than in clinical trials or teaching sessions.

The lack of importance given to the setting up of an appropriate follow-up and removal service can also be judged from the events which followed this training session. In April 1987, a letter from the Family Planning Division of the Thai Ministry of Public Health informed the hospital of a change in policy. Due to its high costs, Norplant would be provided only to specific target groups until further notice, namely "the hilltribes and [other] people living in remote rural areas for whom it is inconvenient to travel to family planning services."

Norplant: a method for population control programmes?

According to the Population Council, the aim of their introduction programme is "to enable developing countries to make new contraceptives available ...with attention to safety, provider competence, easy availability, proper counselling, and follow-up services " (Sivin 1988, p. 81). Our study raises strong doubts about the quality of the training provided in this Thai district hospital.

The incompleteness of medical records and the many missing records are the first indication that the main focus of the training was to pass on the technical skills needed for insertion while neglecting other important aspects of providing Norplant.

These are the other main problems detected:

- Potentially incomplete and/or misleading information to women before insertion;
- Provision of Norplant to women who should not use it because of age or medical history;
- No arrangement for routine medical follow-up;
- No recording of early removals nor reasons for removal;
- No training for removal;
- No system for finding women to remind them of the need for removal after five years.

The intention of this article is not to discredit a particular hospital[2]. We wanted to point out that the Population Council's Norplant Introduction Programme does not automatically result in a high quality service when Norplant is used as a regular method in family planning programmes.

2 This is the reason we are withholding the names of the health professionals who, out of concern for the women's well-being, invited us to do this survey. We want to express our deep gratitude for their invitation and assistance.

Several people within the Population Council, including Senior Research Associate Irving Sivin[3], have referred to the national training in Thailand as an example of the thoroughness of the Population Council's training. However, our findings once again point to what Harvard researcher Donald Warwick describes as "the tension between objectivity and advocacy" within the Population Council. This tension resulted from the organisation's entry into technical assistance. Warwick quotes a Council staff member as saying: "[within the Population Council] there are strong pressures to slant the results towards selling the programme" (Warwick 1982, p. 61-62)[4].

We believe there is an urgent need for an evaluation of training services for the provision of Norplant by independent outside experts, using a client's perspective, before further promoting the introduction of Norplant into national family planning programmes. Our concern is that the introduction of Norplant will produce negative effects, rather than a positive increase in choice of contraceptive methods, when the appropriate service delivery cannot be guaranteed.

References

Leiras Pharmaceuticals *Norplant Contraceptive Implant*. Turku, Finland n.d.

Population Council "Introduction of Norplant and the Copper T 380A IUD: Background For Interagency Meeting." 23-24 March 1988.

Sivin I. "International Experience with Norplant and Norplant-2 contraception". In: *Studies in Family Planning* 1988; (19) 2:81-94.

Warwick Donald P. *Bitter Pills: Population policies and their implementation in eight developing countries.* Cambridge University Press 1982.

3 Irving Sivin, in fact, warns: "It might be anticipated that in countries where the private medical sector has a large role in family planning activities, the organisation of the training programmes may be more spotty and the completeness of physician coverage and the *thoroughness of training* may be less than what has been accomplished in Southeast Asia in the Thai and Indonesian programmes." [our emphasis] (Sivin 1988, p. 93)

4 The main funder of Warwick's study on the actual implementation of family planning programmes, the UNFPA, refused publication when the results turned out to be unsupportive of the official population control policies. The study was therefore published privately.

Bodies of choice: Norplant experimental trials on Egyptian women

by Soheir A. Morsy

"Ask the one who has experience, and not [the one who is] a physician" (Arabic Proverb).

"The development of technology makes it possible for us to make choices about reproduction which were not in our power a short time ago... For any decision there are two kinds of moral issues: one has to do with questions about who should make the decision and the other with what decision ought to be made... First, those who have the power (through control of reproductive technology) to make certain kinds of reproductive decisions – that is, physicians, who are capable of either preventing or enabling people to carry out the technological procedures – do not have a major stake in those decisions. Second, one category of persons that will be crucially affected by reproductive decisions is not only not available for consultation, their existence as persons is contingent on the decision itself" (Sara Ann Ketchum 1987, p. 17, 35).

Introduction

Years prior to the current proliferation of the New Reproductive Technologies, William Shockley, a U.S. Nobel Prize winner in physics, eugenicist and infamous for his advocacy of scientific racism, proposed a programme of cash inducements for sterilisation. Shockley's "scientific" policy recommendation was clearly geared to Black people, and working-class Whites, who tended to have large families, and whose IQ, he asserted, was lower than their middle-class counterparts. The cash inducements were linked by a sliding scale to the person's IQ score (Rose 1976). As for the technology that would support this form of scientific racism, Shockley envisioned the development of "a subcutaneous injection of a contraceptive time capsule which provides a slow seepage of contraceptive hormones until it is removed" (Rose and Hamner 1976).

Shockley's "contraceptive time capsule" is now a reality, distributed under the trademark "Norplant". Prior to the 1990 FDA approval of Norplant for use in the U.S., where it was created, this five-year contraceptive was tested on women in a number of other countries (Population Information Program 1987). For the most part trials have been conducted on women in Asia, the Pacific, Latin America and Africa, notably Egypt, the focus of this account of Norplant experimental trials.

For Egyptian women, as for others, human rights, and, by extension, health, are interwoven into the fabric of social power relations which transcend clinical settings. This paper describes the international socio-political context of Norplant's introduction into Egypt, including development aid and state policies. The promotion of long-term contraception in Egypt is introduced as an illustration of a more general pattern of international fertility regulation.

There has been opposition to Norplant's introduction within the Egyptian professional medical community. Some affiliates of the prestigious faculties of medicine at Cairo and Alexandria Universities, as well as other professors of medicine, have expressed reservations about Norplant, or outright opposition to the trials of Norplant and of other forms of long-term contraception. These opinions are presented in the second section of this paper. They stand in contrast to the much publicised opinions of Norplant researchers and promoters, and derivative press accounts.

Following an overview of these critical opinions, I present an account of the role of the media based on a survey of the Egyptian national press, including the opposition press, over the past decade. This covers the period of experimental trials of the "miracle capsule", leading up to its approval for general use by the Ministry of Health in 1989.

The next major section focuses on Egyptian women as "bodies of choice" for these trials. In 1985, during a one week consultancy visit to Assiut University's Department of Obstetrics and Gynaecology, I conducted interviews of women taking part in trials of Norplant, and medical staff at Assiut University's family planning clinic. This was the site of one of Egypt's four centres of contraceptive implant research. This consultancy visit was initiated by the Population Council's Cairo Regional Office in order to determine the feasibility of a sociomedical study of Norplant contraception. (Morsy 1985).

The "time capsule" and international modernist development

On first impression one may think that the present setting and ideological framework for the use of contraceptive implants are basically different from those associated with Schockley's scheme. Unlike the "time capsule", Norplant is not confined to the U.S.; clinical trials have been conducted all over the world. Neither is Shockley's blatant form of racism associated with Norplant introduction in the Third World. Nevertheless, Norplant, as a surgically implantable/removable, provider-dependent technology approximates Shockley's vision in that it harbours an inherent potential for the imposition of biomedically-mediated social control over women's reproductive capacities. But unlike the explicit intent associated with Shockley's "time capsule", Norplant's introduction within the framework of existing global power relations may well serve as a "back door to eugenics" (Duster 1990).

The envisioned "time capsule" technology-turned-real is linked to a seemingly desirable form of social engineering. Norplant was introduced to the Third World within the framework of modernisation/development programmes. Its population control, as opposed to family planning function (Amin 1976) was, and is, veiled by its promotion as a "modern medical method" or a locally valued form of "technology transfer" from an industrialised country. This type of symbol manipulation is particularly effective when the new contraceptive technology is transferred within the framework of international programmes for scientific cooperation. The illusion of enhanced development potential bestowed by allegedly objective, ethically-neutral science obscures the political implications of such cooperation (Badran 1984; El-Bayoumi 1982; Dickson 1984).

Beyond the all too familiar rationalisations of the international development establishment (Escobar 1988), consideration of what Sylvia Noble Tesh describes as the "hidden arguments" of dominant medical ideas (Noble Tesh 1989) exposes international population control ideology as an expression of global power relations. This ideology presents a single aspect of reality and obscures its relation to others, notably the social origins of the need for large families. Thus, neglect befalls state and international policies which prevent equitable distribution of resources or a system of power sharing which would include women as equal partners. Given the social significance of large families, women's "forgetfulness" in taking the pill, which Norplant is designed to overcome, may be nothing less than a form of "women's everyday resistance" against state-sanctioned population control efforts (Hammami and Rieker 1988).

The technological fix remains a key element of international population control programmes within a global framework of acute differences in power. Illustrations of what has been described as "the dark side of contraceptive 'choice'" (Shapiro 1985), which compromise human dignity, continue to occur. Contraceptive methods for women are often promoted without attention to necessary precautions, in spite of the proven dangers of certain devices or in the absence of convincing evidence of long-term safety (Yanoshik and Norsigian 1989).

Development aid and population control in Egypt

Within the framework of Egypt's current "openness" to imported development expertise, the country has witnessed persistent international support for population control programmes. The U.S. government, in particular, either directly through its USAID (United States Agency for International Development) Cairo mission, or indirectly through such agencies as the International Planned Parenthood Federation, provides the Egyptian government with ample funding for birth control. Foreign assistance extends to "private sector family planning" (Mokhtar 1989). Furthermore, between 1975 and 1983 over half (51.5%) of the total U.S. budgetary allocation for Egyptian health development was allocated for population control programmes (Galal 1988).

International efforts to curtail Egypt's high birth rate have been relentless, including pressure from the World Bank (Kaplan 1976) and threats from AID officials "not to give more aid [sic]" (Lalevee 1982; Morsy 1986a). The latter have repeatedly stated their dedication to curtailing Egyptian population growth, an effort which has been described by one of them, Mr. Lennie Kangas, as analogous to operating on a cancer (Dickey 1986). Such determination has also been expressed in the same breath as racist remarks of alleged "deep-seated cultural failure throughout the [Egyptian] population to relate cause and effect" (Ibid).

In 1982, Egypt's new president extended his personal support to curbing population growth (Kennedy 1986). The National Population Council, chaired by the president himself, replaced Egypt's National Family Planning Commission. Remarking on the failure of the Family Planning Commission to address the country's population problem, USAID's Mr Mario Jaramillo criticised its head, Dr Aziz El-Bindari, for taking "precious family-planning funds and [spending] them on development as well" (MacKenzie 1985). Not unlike many other Egyptian colleagues (El-Issawi 1985), Dr. El-Bindari believes that economic development is itself the best contraceptive.

The controversy surrounding the introduction of Norplant in Egypt

In 1984, Dr. Maher Mahran, a gynaecologist, and prominent member of the ruling National Democratic Party, took charge of the National Population Council. In 1985 he announced that he intended to prevent "economic progress [from being] cancelled out by the demands of increasing population". In expressing his support for new, long-lasting contraceptive technologies he went on to state that Norplant has been tested on 2,000 Egyptian women, with good results" and that it "will be tested on 10,000 more as soon as supplies of the implants become available" (MacKenzie 1985). The opinions of the targets of this programme of "modern science", the poor women of Egypt, have not been included in the very limited public discussion surrounding the introduction of Norplant.

Norplant was introduced in Egypt within the framework of international scientific cooperation. Professor Mamdouh Shaaban, an active promoter of the implant and a professor at the Faculty of Medicine at Assiut University, explained the role of Egypt at the 1984 International Symposium on Long-term Subdermal Contraceptive Implants. He stated that "Egypt was the first African nation to take part in the international effort to test the acceptability of Norplant". He went on to assert that "due consideration" had been given to the safety of the method by the Egyptian Ministry of Health before approving clinical trials (Shaaban 1984). This claim has been challenged by other physicians who have seriously considered the issue of long-term safety. In the same conference proceedings, a team of researchers from Alexandria University's Faculty of Medicine expressed conditional support for the implant:

> "[Norplant]...may have a place in family planning programmes, especially if long-term research indicates its total safety... the subdermal implants regimen could be expected to suit some users and to be rejected by others" (El-Sahwi et al. 1984).

In a public testimony on amenorrhoea, documented as a side effect of both Norplant and Depo Provera [another long-acting progestin-only contraceptive], a member of the same Alexandria team, Professor Toppozada, provided medically-informed commentary which contrasts with the convenient framing of contraception-induced cessation of menstruation as medically unimportant. At the U.S. House of Representatives' Select Committee Hearings on Populations, Professor Toppozada stated that the health consequences of cycle alterations among women with endemic diseases, which are prevalent among rural Egyptian women, or metabolic disorders, was an unresolved question. His testimony revealed "[the] paucity of information regarding any metabolic disturbances or hormonal changes related to prolonged amenorrhoea" (Toppozada as cited in Rakusen 1981, p. 88).

Some Egyptian physicians have expressed objection to the very principle of clinical trials on Egyptian women, whether in relation to Norplant or to Depo Provera. Professor Aziz Khattab of Ain-Shams University's Faculty of Medicine reiterated his Cairo University colleagues' strong opposition to the use of the latter. Refusing to allow the Egyptian people to be turned into "experimental animals", he stated,

> "Let America experiment with these injections in America, but for them to be tested in Egypt, we refuse this..." (*Tabibak El-Khas*, December 1985, p. 17)

Cognisant of the fact that the original Norplant research had been conducted in the U.S., and that Upjohn, the company which distributes Depo Provera, is also U.S.-based, Egyptian physicians have objected to the introduction of these contraceptives in the absence of their approval by the U.S. Food and Drug Administration (FDA). Remarking on the international double standard, Professor Gamal El-Kholi, of Tanta University's Faculty of Medicine, noted in the Egyptian monthly *Tabibak al-Khas* [Your private Physician] that:

> "In the U.S. the use of Depo Provera as a contraceptive is not approved, yet Depo Provera is distributed in the Third World... In Egypt, about three months ago, the U.S. Agency for Aid decided to give the National Population Council $3 million to spend on the subcutaneous capsules... which [contain] progestogen... and cause the same side-effects as Depo Provera; besides, the method is still under experimentation... To protect the health of... women and mothers, all experiments conducted on the injections and the subcutaneous capsules should be stopped until their effectiveness without side effects is proven" (*Tabibak El-Khas* December 1985, pp. 19-20).

Attempts to popularise the controversy surrounding Norplant trials, such as that illustrated by *Tabibak El-Khas*, remained exceptional (Morsy 1986b, 1986c). Most of the concerns about Norplant have been voiced at professional meetings. In contrast, proponents of Norplant, backed by official sanction, have practically monopolised the Egyptian mass media. As a result, the administrators of the National Population Council stood accused of forfeiting the Council's mission in favour of "mere propaganda for [selected contraceptive] devices". Commenting on the "directing of the mass media to focus on personal acclaim rather than serious field work", the editor of *Tabibak El-Khas* added that:

> "[it is] not logical to expect... millions of families in villages and hamlets to sit around television sets to listen to the 'group of four' [medical professionals] presenting a unified opinion in closed meetings [for] complicated scientific entertainment" (*Tabibak El-Khas* December 1985, p. 13).

The "magic capsule" in the national press

The national press has played an active role in the promotion of Norplant as a contraceptive. Although the majority of women who are targeted for this type of birth control are illiterate, they are influenced by promotional articles in the press through literate members of their communities (Morsy, 1985). In general, the press has hailed Norplant as a major technological advance, even describing it as "the magic capsule" (*Al-Ahram* February 2, 1984). Downplaying, or even denying Norplant's known side effects, ignoring the social implications of the need for surgical removal of the implant, and assuring its "total" safety in the absence of studies of its long-term effects, some press evaluations have gone beyond enthusiastic support to the point of deception (*Al-Ahram* February 23, 24 and 25, 1984; March 5, 1985. *Al Akhbar* March 8, 18, 1984; April 4,18, 1985. *Akhbar El-Yom* March 2, 1985).

Consistent with the official position, the state-regulated press has tended to single out women's procreative capacities as an impediment to development, resorting to visual representations in the form of sexist cartoons to propagate this idea.[1] The press has given prominence to the opinions of university professors who strongly support long-term subdermal contraception. Relatively neglected is the above noted more guarded support expressed by the research team from Alexandria University's Faculty of Medicine.

An exceptional mention of the rejection of Norplant by a Kasr-El-Aini professor of medicine appeared in the national press in 1981 (*Al-Ahram* June 24, 1981). However, only an opposition party newspaper elaborated the health risks which prompted this physician's rejection. Under the heading "The Poor Women of Egypt: Experimental Mice for America", the paper demanded an

1 During the month of January, 1989, in particular, *Al-Ahram* published a series of such cartoons. This coincided with the appearance of a number of articles pertaining to fertility regulation, and more importantly, the announcement by the Ministry of Health permitting the general use of Norplant.

explanation of the effects of this experimentation on the health of Egyptian women (*Al-Shaab* August 4, 1981). None was provided by the Ministry of Health.

With national press claims of Norplant's safety continuing unabated, Egyptians read praises of the "magic capsule" including the ease and painlessness of its insertion, free of charge. This occurred in the absence of clarification of how women had "volunteered" for contraceptive experimentation, nor mention of any difficulty facing a woman's access to the "simple surgical procedure [of removal].. at any time [she] wants" (*Al-Akhbar* March 18, April 4, 1985).

To support its claims of safety, the Egyptian press has made reference to international bodies such as the World Health Organization (WHO), international scientists, and Egyptian Norplant researchers. Examination of WHO's relevant memorandum contradicted the assertion that this U.N. agency has affirmed Norplant's safety (*Akhbar El-Yom* March 2, 1985). To the contrary, the WHO 1985 memorandum stated that "there have, as yet, been no epidemiological studies of long-term safety" (WHO 1985, p. 487, 491). In this regard it is worth noting that among the members of the consultation group who drafted the WHO memorandum were individuals with clear vested interest in Norplant research and the marketing of the contraceptive. These included representatives from the Population Council, the research centre which developed Norplant, and Huhtamaki Oy/Leiras Pharmaceuticals of Finland, which manufactures Norplant under license from the Population Council. Among the list of memorandum signatories was also the name of the same Egyptian physician/Norplant researcher who has been favoured by national press coverage of his evaluations of Norplant, including the assertion of "absence of any side effects" (*Al-Akhbar* March 8, 1984).

Resorting to the manipulation of culturally meaningful symbols of "progress", "modernity", and "development", the national press has encouraged Egyptian women to follow "international" contraception trends, noting the official approval of Norplant in Finland and anticipated licensing in the U.S.[2] The concern with "modernity" ignores the differences between poor and undernourished Egyptian women and their relatively affluent counterparts in Scandinavia where Norplant has been approved as a contraceptive (Kunstadter 1980). As for the press' reference to the long anticipated [U.S.] FDA approval of Norplant, even this regulatory agency's determination of

2 The U.S. is the epitome of the western way of life, which is held up as ideal within the framework of Egypt's current orientation of "emulation and dependence" (Abdel Fadil 1989).

"safety" is not to be accepted uncritically. This is illustrated by a National Women's Health Network report released to the U.S. Congress (Haire 1984), and the more recent medical concerns which followed FDA approval [discussed on page 108-109].

The Egyptian press has also continued to ignore the potential for abuse of this provider-dependent contraceptive in light of the marked power differential between Norplant research subjects and family planning physicians in Egypt. Within the framework of another form of ideological manipulation, which favours the privatisation of family planning services, the press *itself* has exposed the less than humane treatment of female patrons of public family planning clinics at the hands of clinic medical staff (Mokhtar 1989).

Illustrative of the less than kind treatment of rural women at public health clinics is a commentary by anthropologist Hania Sholkamy based on fieldwork in Upper Egypt. Referring to several women "who have been subject to [Norplant] contraception without having been informed of the possible side-effects" she documents the reaction of a physician to the women's suffering. In response to the anthropologist's observation that a woman was experiencing blackouts, severe loss in weight and delayed menstruation following the insertion of the capsules, the physician "expressed no alarm or sentiment, saying that all forms of contraception had side effects". Far from feeling concern for the women who use Norplant, this physician saw that "the important thing for the government and for the country as a whole was to reduce the number of births" (Sholkamy 1988, p. 149).

Following a period of much more limited reference to Norplant in the national press, a January 1989 report on "a new method of contraception" (*Al-Ahram* January 5, 1989) provided a less exaggerated version of the "benefits" of Norplant than earlier press accounts. In addition to presenting the implant as one among a number of available contraceptives, the report refers to side effects. However, similar to earlier accounts, it asserts that the capsule "can be removed at any time a woman wants", a claim contradicted by the testimony of Norplant users themselves (Morsy 1985). Although reference is made to side effects in this more recent press account, this is accompanied by the assurance that Norplant "does not affect the woman's ability to carry out her daily work". The validity of this claim is in turn challenged by direct observations (Hania Sholkamy, personal communication, 1987).

In the same article, the reference to follow-up visits to a physician is contradicted by the accompanying impression that Norplant is maintenance free. It is suggested that once the capsule is inserted, "there is nothing asked of [the woman] except to remember one date, the date when the capsule is to be removed". In clear contradiction to the WHO directive for medical surveillance (1985), this opinion is confirmed by Dr Eiz-el-Din Osman, professor of Obstetrics and Gynaecology and Executive Director of the Egyptian Fertility Association, which distributes the implants to clinics. He is quoted as stating that Norplant "overcomes, among others, the problem of forgetfulness of taking pills by mouth... the woman has the Norplant inserted, then she forgets it for five years". Moreover, while there *is* reference to contraindications, the "basic facts about the device" *do not* mention the recommendation against use during breast feeding. This is no minor omission in light of the prevalence of nursing among Egyptian mothers.

Biomedical versus user perspectives

During the consultancy visit to Assiut I interviewed the members of the medical staff of the University's Family Planning Clinic. In the same clinic I met about fifty women with Norplant implants. Outside of the Assiut clinic, I interviewed a group of ten implant users in their homes, in town and in two nearby villages. Women's opinions about the use of implants were also gleaned from the attendants of a state health unit in one of these villages.

In addition to the limited duration of the consultancy period, my attempt to document women's evaluations of Norplant was constrained by the almost constant presence of medical personnel during my encounters with women in the clinic. This extended to encounters with women in their homes, to which members of the family planning clinic staff also escorted me.[3] Nevertheless, meeting with women who have at one time or another experienced implant contraception, and those close to them, yielded evaluations which contrasted with biomedical pronouncements regarding "acceptability" and "satisfaction".

Beyond its courteous and professional tenor, my encounters with biomedical personnel during my consultancy visit to Assiut University yielded evaluations of Norplant which differed from those of the press accounts noted above. The researchers readily discussed Norplant's known side effects and the limited effectiveness of their medical interventions. The latter amounted to no more than the prescription of "tonics" for symptomatic relief. As for the difference in power between themselves and their clients, the physicians denied that this difference affected the ability of women to exercise informed choice about contraceptives. Yet, the physicians reasoned that it was difficult

---

3 My inquiry was free of this surveillance when I interviewed people on the street during walks around town and in the bazaar area. Similarly unrestricted was an interview conducted with a female gynaecologist who is not affiliated with Assiut University.

to explain to women how Norplant worked since they were "uneducated", or, as one physician put it, their understanding was "very limited".

The physicians' own judgement of what is an appropriate contraceptive was described as a scientifically-based recommendation. The priority of clinical judgement was further rationalised by reference to a Contraception Screening Check List. This form is intended to document medically relevant criteria for determining who is eligible for Norplant contraception and is based on the results of a pelvic examination and socio-demographic characteristics of potential Norplant "acceptors". In response to my inquiry about possible long-term adverse effects of implant contraception, the clinic staff referred to a monitoring plan involving a series of scheduled visits to the clinic.

Consistent with a clinic physician's observation of my readily acknowledged "bias" towards women, I explicitly commented that I was concerned with women's health, not the promotion of contraception, during the first meeting with the clinic patrons.[4] Not expecting that members of the biomedical staff would continue to be present, I also promised to convey the women's grievances to the clinic staff. The questions I asked the women covered several topics of concern. I asked about their reasons for accepting Norplant; how they heard about it, who introduced them to the clinic, their husband's role in their decision to use Norplant and prior contraceptive use. I also asked about the health effects of Norplant, notably menstrual irregularities, the health implications for their children, specifically for nursing infants, perceived side effects and their treatment, the effect of Norplant on sexual relations, follow-up visits to the clinic, reasons for continuation or removal, as well as the role of physicians in advising women on continuation and termination. Understandably, under conditions of collective interviewing and the constant presence of clinic personnel, women responded to some questions and avoided others. Some women also responded to me non-verbally and others replied secretly at opportune moments, for example when they hugged me or shook my hand at the end of the meeting.

The meetings with women revealed that their knowledge of Norplant contraception was influenced by the mass media. In addition, some had first become interested in the implants after conversations with other users, including allegedly paid recruiters for the family planning clinic. In the presence of medical personnel a number of women at the clinic, particularly those who have used Norplant for up to four years, eagerly expressed their

4 The Family Planning Clinic had mailed letters to most of these women instructing them to visit the clinic during the consultancy period.

great satisfaction, some referring positively to associated weight gain. In response to my own questioning, and encouragement, some of the very women who articulated Norplant's advantages also expressed apprehension about its long-term effects on themselves or on their nursing infants. Women also described various aches and pains, in addition to nausea, dizziness, bloating, and headaches. Much of their concern was focused on menstrual irregularities ranging from amenorrhoea to spotting, and heavy bleeding, which they referred to with the Arabic term for haemorrhaging.

In contrast to the guarded responses to my questions by women at the family planning clinic, those interviewed in two nearby villages, particularly those visited in their homes, spoke of their suffering much more freely. In addition to noting the familiar side effects, including menstrual disturbances, they referred to depression and weight loss. Some also openly expressed anger at the family planning clinic physicians for their repeated refusal to remove the capsules. Outside the clinic, some of them confronted the physicians who accompanied me, charging their senior colleagues with refusal to remove the implants.

Of the six detailed accounts given to me by women who encountered difficulties in having the implant removed, the following three summaries are provided as illustrations:

Shalabiya's experience

Shalabiya [pseudonym] said that she had the capsules inserted four years and seven months earlier. She complained that they were making her sick and weak. She explained that if she had been stronger she would have had lots of children, but she was not and that is why she had the capsules inserted. But instead of preserving her strength they had made her sick. She went to the doctor to have them removed when they began to bother her several months after insertion but he refused. Her menstrual irregularity, about which she complained to the doctor, continued for nine months. At the time she suffered from what she described as severe "haemorrhaging".

After the first nine months her periods became regular again, but the problem started again six months prior to our interview. Shalabiya said that she had "all the symptoms but no period". She went to see a doctor who prescribed medicine, but to no avail. Upon my request for clarification, she explained that she had told the same doctor who had inserted the capsules in her arm that she wanted them removed, but he refused again. Shalabiya said that she had tried to see the doctor again, sometimes as often as twice a month, but she was always told that he was away. She believed that the clinic personnel were just stalling her. Referring to the side effects of Norplant, she said, "one might as well have a child. Either I have a child and be uncomfortable, or use a contraceptive and be uncomfortable". She also pointed out that her husband had been away for two years and that she had no use for the capsules anyway. This, in her opinion, was all the more reason for the physician to remove the capsules.

Shalabiya's reasoning has implications beyond her specific case. The male migration pattern in her village as a whole prompts one to question the appropriateness of implant contraception for women whose husbands are absent from the country for extended periods of time, and among whom extra-marital sexual intercourse is a most unlikely practice.[5]

Amira's determination to have the capsules removed

Amira [pseudonym] had the implant inserted four years prior to the interview. She reported suffering from amenorrhoea for the first nine months following insertion. At the time she also suffered from general fatigue, dizziness and headache. She nursed her infant for only a short time before her milk dried up. Her menstrual cycle started, and irregular bleeding continued for weeks. Six months prior to the interview "haemorrhaging" started and continued for weeks. She went to see the doctor at the family planning clinic to have the capsules removed, after a number of visits to him in pursuit of "relief". The doctor simply refused. He tried to assure her that she would improve and that the problem was transient. Upon failure to get his consent, she resorted to a doctor outside of the family planning clinic who had established a practice in the vicinity of her village. He removed the capsules for a fee of seven pounds, as a favour to her husband. She became pregnant after the removal of Norplant.

One of the physicians from the family planning clinic who was present during my visit to Amira's home checked her scar and declared it "fine". Amira expressed rage at the doctors of the Assiut University Family Planning Clinic but had very kind words for the doctor who removed the implant, describing him as her "saviour".

Bahana's decision to remove the implant

Bahana [pseudonym] had originally heard about the capsules from two other women in her village. In the interview which I conducted with her before the removal of the implants, and after her surgery, which I observed, she recounted that she had had the capsules for two years before she decided to have them removed. She explained that she had felt fine for

---

5 In a study of Shalabiya's village, anthropologist Nicholas Hopkins (1985) estimates between 250 and 300 men were working abroad in 1981. He notes that the migrants were "mature men... with a wife and children at home."

the first eight months, but had suffered from severe bleeding for four months afterwards. She said that her bleeding had been so heavy that she had used four towels every day.

In dealing with the problem Bahana went to see two doctors in her village and asked to have the capsules removed. Both physicians refused and reportedly said, "have the person who put them in remove them". Although it was a university affiliated physician who had inserted the capsules for her in his private hospital in Assiut, she first asked the physicians in the village where she lived because of transportation and time limitations. She said that she was poor and had to help her husband to earn a living. The day of her surgery she had to leave her village at six o'clock in the morning in order to arrive in time at ll a.m. for the removal of the capsules at the University Hospital in Assiut. Regarding her husband's reaction to her "haemorrhaging", she said that he was furious because she was depleted of energy. She agreed with my suggestion that the bleeding's interference with sexual intercourse also angered her husband. In the course of our conversation this poor, illiterate peasant woman shared with me her fear of surgery and her worry that she would be charged for the removal of the capsules. She said that she had paid what was, in fact, an incredibly large sum of money to have the capsules inserted by a private physician.

The personal experiences of these women obviously contradict "the state's slogan which condemns subjugation and forced use [of contraception]... [and favours] consciousness raising" (*Al-Ahram* September 1, 1987). Beyond specific cases, my encounters with Norplant users generally presented a sharp contrast to the mass media allegations of a lack of side effects. While some women repeated physicians' praises of Norplant and noted their willingness to "endure" the side effects in order to avoid pregnancy, others announced their reservations, complaints, and in some cases outright rage. In addition to the above-noted discomforts, women reported distress associated with a perception that Norplant-induced amenorrhoea resulted in the accumulation of "poison" in the body. Some women expressed a general fear of the physical consequences of a foreign object inserted in the arm, and a specific concern with "the bad disease" (cancer). Women also pointed to the threat of divorce from husbands who were not willing to tolerate the prolonged bleeding which they believed caused women to feel tired and which could also result in forced abstention from sexual intercourse.

Women's concerns about the health consequences of Norplant extended to its effects on their breast-fed children. While some women said that the capsule increased their supply of breast milk, others believed that it dried it up and forced mothers to switch to "artificial nursing". Unaware that

Norplant was not recommended for nursing mothers, a patient of the family planning clinic was visibly upset when she heard me state this restriction. She had just had Norplant inserted and accused the clinic staff of not informing her of the restriction for nursing. In desperation, this woman turned to me and said that for herself she is "willing to endure the capsules, but what about the child, what is his sin?"

My encounters, outside the clinic, with some of the residents of Assiut also shed light on local perceptions of Norplant. In these relatively unrestricted conversations, the evaluations made by women and men whom I met on the streets and in the bazaar of this Upper Egyptian town contrasted with the "success" story purveyed by the media. A vocal, literate opponent expressed suspicion of the "capsule experiment" and the use of poor women as "experimental animals". Another man referred to the mass media's "fooling the uneducated women". A professional woman who did not use Norplant described how women had been herded, "like cattle", to the clinic and how some women functioned as "contractors" to recruit others in return for payment. Regarding the clinic's check list, this evaluative instrument was judged as "ink on paper". Sarcasm was also expressed about the duty of clinic staff to inform women about breast-feeding as grounds for exclusion and their responsibility to carry out a pelvic examination prior to insertion.

Acceptability, continuity, and safety in context

Medical studies of Norplant "acceptors" in Egypt either ignore the issue of informed consent or assert women's acceptance. For example, a study in Zagazig simply states that women "gave their consent to use the new method after receiving due explanation" (Said et al. 1984). Given the acknowledged difficulty of "communication" between physicians and their illiterate patients, the meaning of "due explanation" requires due clarification.

Considering the bombardment of women with distorted media accounts, physicians' elitist attitudes towards "uneducated" women, and the absence of effective institutions for the protection of health care consumers, not to mention human subjects in experimental trials, one is left with serious concerns about the meaning of "volunteering" for clinical trials and "acceptance" of contraceptive implants by underprivileged women. In the Egyptian context in which Norplant contraception has been introduced, women confront professional medical control without even the benefit of the type of "defensive medicine" that is practised by physicians in the technology-exporting country as a result of a fear of malpractice lawsuits (Dobson 1986). More fundamental is the framework of power relations which allows what physicians themselves have described as women's "tolerance of the menstrual irregularities to an extent that surpassed initial expectations" (Shaaban and Salah 1984, p. 26).

In contrast to officially-sanctioned efforts of promoting Norplant "acceptability", discussions of safety have remained confined to specialised academic journals or international research conferences. The implant users whom I met in Assiut were certainly not informed of the implications of research carried out at Assiut University. Significant in this regard is a study published in the University's *Proceedings of the Symposium on Long-term Contraceptive Implants.* The authors state that "the mean gains in body weight and length of the infants of the mothers using Norplant were significantly lower than those in infants of other... control groups" (Salem et al. 1984, p. 140).

Also in relation to acceptability, Norplant researchers claim that the implant is culturally suitable as it "may suit very much our rural women who are careless in taking the daily pill and who are usually afraid of using the IUD". In the same vein it is argued that "some of them are shy to be exposed to gynaecological examinations" (Said et al. 1984, p. 29). Another Norplant researcher highlights the rationalisation that "injection in the arm avoids the mortifying experience of exposing one's genitals to medical scrutiny" (Salah 1983, p. 4).

Beyond the appeal of apparent sensitivity to local women's modesty, the alleged cultural compatibility of Norplant is in direct contradiction to physicians' own declared commitment to "medical scrutiny", including a pelvic examination prior to insertion of the implant. When health is a priority that can only be met through "exposing one's genitals to medical scrutiny" (WHO 1985, p. 491), avoidance of gynaecological examinations for cultural reasons can clearly reduce safety. In practice, however, the high value that women place on health often prompts them to side-step certain cultural prescriptions, "shyness" included.

In addition, the safety requirement for close medical surveillance of Norplant users contradicts the impression that it is convenient because it is maintenance free. Insuring safety through regular follow-up medical exams limits the alleged "put it in and forget it" advantages of Norplant. Beyond stereotypical characterisations of "our rural women", who are said to be "careless in taking the daily pill", women may also be "forgetful" of their follow-up medical exams. This is likely to be the case given their numerous responsibilities and the unenticing atmosphere of family planning clinics. If safety is indeed a primary consideration, then Norplant contraception requires *special* maintenance rather than no maintenance.

The statistical data provided by Norplant researchers on the high rates of satisfaction among users also deserves critical evaluation. A study presented at the Assiut International Symposium states that by the end of the second year after insertion, of the group of "original acceptors of Norplant", "eighty-eight percent of them rated it as good or excellent and the rest as unfavourable or bad (Shaaban 1984, p. 25). In light of some women's reports of physicians insisting that they "hold on", such ratings cannot be accepted at face value. Such statistical data hide the stress endured by women who are confronted by the refusal of Norplant researchers to remove the implant.

Regardless of the validity of specific charges that physicians refused to remove Norplant, whether in Egypt or elsewhere (Reis n.d; UBINIG 1988)[6], implant contraception undoubtedly increases physicians' control over women's reproductive capacities. This was clearly demonstrated during my encounter with a Norplant user in her home, accompanied by two physicians from the Family Planning Clinic of Assiut University. The user complained about a clinic physician's refusal to remove the implants. She added, "if they refuse again I will go outside (the Family Planning Clinic/University system)". One of the physicians in our company defiantly replied, "you cannot".

In addition to blatant challenges of this type and women's endurance of physical discomfort, statistical data showing high continuation rates conceal the threats of husbands who disapprove of implant contraception. In sum, the construction of "satisfaction" outside of its personal or social context, with its focus on "how many", even if statistically credible, eclipses how women have come to "tolerate" Norplant to an extent that surpassed the expectations of Norplant researchers themselves.

Conclusion: beyond the medical provider – user divide

> *"... there continues to be colonization of a different kind which women of colour in the United States, Black women in Britain and women in "third world" countries have identified and struggled against... The location of western feminists within an existing hierarchy of power between "first world" and "third world" countries, with differential/preferential access to funding, publishing houses, organising international conferences, and so on, help to subordinate*

---

6 Copies of both of these works were kindly shared with me by Dr Amal Abdel Hadi, a co-member of the Egyptian Association For Health and Environmental Development (AHED).

and often erase the political struggles of "third world" women" (Jacqui Alexander 1990:53).

> *"The language of options is seductive because it sounds so much like freedom and mutual respect. Even feminists fall for it... But F.D.A. hearings [on breast implants] show where the refusal to analyze the actual content of individual decisions ends up: in mutilated bodies... The next time medicine comes up with a cure for the "disease" of being female, let's let guinea pigs be the guinea pigs"* (Katha Pollitt 1992:329).

Most of the concerns over the abuse of Norplant contraception addressed in this paper were expressed in my 1985 consultancy report to the Population Council and Assiut University's Department of Obstetrics and Gynaecology. This report, submitted over seven years ago, has not yet been made accessible to the public. On my part, in keeping with the ethical code of my profession, and with the support of my anthropologist colleagues and other human rights and health activists, I have maintained my resolve to publicise the contents of the report. In doing so, I have been confronted by the gate-keeping tactics of the population and feminist establishments, including a publicly articulated charge of "sensationalism", and the limiting of women's contraceptive "choice". Needless to say, this is not a unique experience for those of us who are committed to challenge hegemonic wisdom, whether it takes the form of authoritative medical "science" (Price 1992), discourse on reproductive "choice" (Davis 1990; Alvarez Martinez 1992) or scholarly expressions of the "White Man's[/Woman's] Burden" (Mani 1990; Mohanty 1984; Morsy 1991).

At first glance it might be concluded that the issues surrounding the technological management of reproduction in Egypt bear no resemblance to those affecting women in the industrially developed U.S., where Norplant originated and where it is now promoted. To the contrary, beyond the specific differences noted below, Jacqui Alexander's "colonization of a different kind" becomes important at the level of "determinate mechanisms" (Leacock 1972). The proponents of "individual choice" as reproductive rights remove reproduction from its wider social context. (E. Martinez 1992) In contrast, identification of shared "colonization" requires nothing short of rejection of the desocialised view of individual choice. (Martin 1988).

Unlike self-manageable contraception which is promoted by feminist groups in the industrially developed world (NWHN 1988), long term, provider-dependent methods are favoured by the international population control establishment. This is deemed particularly suitable for Third World women, as it is for ethnic minorities, mentally retarded women, and incarcerated women in the U.S., who allegedly cannot practice contraception responsibly (BWHC 1984).

In the U.S., around the time of withdrawal of FDA support for breast implants, the mass media judiciously proceeded with the "manufacturing of consent" [to borrow Naom Chomsky's phraseology] for another type of implant, Norplant. Favourable mass media accounts of Norplant presented it as eagerly pursued by women of an ethnic minority [Latinas in Dallas County] (*ABC Nightly News* April 13, 1991), and called it "painless and invisible" (*Mademoiselle* June 1991), as well as "highly effective", "highly acceptable" (*Working Mother* February 1990), and "not susceptible to user error" (*Time* January 21, 1991). It was also described as "a birth-control breakthrough", and "totally reversible (Cowley 1990).

Similar to the Egyptian press' assurance of safety by referring to Norplant's approval in Finland, favourable U.S. press accounts of Norplant assert its safety by stating that it has "already [been] approved [in 16 other countries]", and "tested in more than 500,000 volunteers worldwide". It is also suggested that "Women in Finland and Sweden had no trouble getting used to the device,... nor did their counterparts in Indonesia or Bangladesh". Illustrative of the minimisation of the side effect of menstrual disruption is a quote from a Norplant researcher who considers "the abnormal bleeding [as] usually too light to require even a sanitary napkin and that it diminishes with time" (Cowley 1990).

Beyond the praise of Norplant, including repeated reference to the culturally significant notion of enhanced individual choice, and related deriding of the "birth control backlash" (Hilts 1990), the U.S. mass media, unlike its Egyptian counterpart, has been, at once, instrumental in bringing attention to the implant's limitations. Notable in this regard are Norplant's questionable long-term safety and the potential for abuse of this provider-dependent technology (*Glamour* June 1991; Hilts 1990; Purvis 1990). Such reservations had been expressed by feminists/health activists prior to the 1990 FDA approval of Norplant for contraceptive use in the U.S. (NWHN 1989).

Regarding the social status of U.S. women targeted for Norplant contraception, its resemblance to that of their Egyptian counterparts is inescapable. Consistent with Shockley's original scheme for social control, U.S. welfare mothers have been proposed as bodies of choice for implant contraception. *The Philadelphia Inquirer*'s much publicised suggestion that "black welfare recipients should be offered money to use [Norplant]" (*Newsweek* December 31, 1990) is certainly reminiscent of Shockley's vision. So are some state officials' proposals of public subsidies and monetary incentives for Norplant insertion (ACLU 1992; Kansas House Bill 2089 as cited in ACLU, 1991; Murray 1992; *San Francisco Chronicle* May 17, 1991). Consistent with the long-term support of the U.S. upper class for population control efforts (Shapiro 1985) "philanthropists" have recently become involved in a Baltimore based campaign to promote Norplant among teenage women "... in some of the city's poorest neighbourhoods" (*Washington Post* December 4, 1992).

The targeting of low income women has prompted protest from the ACLU [American Civil Liberties Union]. Activists working with the ACLU's Reproductive Freedom Project have exposed the inherent race bias of the proposed public programmes, and "Norplant's unprecedented characteristics to lock women into contraceptive choices they might not otherwise make" (ACLU 1991). Warnings of potential Norplant abuse have also come from African-American feminists/health activists (Baker 1991; Ferris 1991), the Native [American] Women's Reproductive Rights Coalition, and the National Latina Health Organisation. Expressions of concern in the U.S. extend to biomedical professionals, including bioethicists and physicians (Gladwell 1990; Lewin 1991). In a 1990 letter to the editor of the *Washington Post* a physician wrote:

> "I am dismayed that Norplant is being touted as a contraceptive that "advances freedom and responsibility"... Protection against pregnancy is not the only consideration... Norplant offers no protection whatsoever against the AIDS virus... Although there is no doubt that effective and safe contraception... is needed, this should not detract us from raising basic questions about the conditions under which new forms of contraception are developed, tested and used" (El-Bayoumi 1990).

More recently the American Medical Association has condemned judges who sentence women to use Norplant (*Washington Post* December 4, 1992).

As in Egypt, the issue of Norplant's safety remains contestable among U.S. medical professionals even after FDA approval of the contraceptive. The assertion of the implant's safety because it contains "one of the hormones in oral contraceptives" (*Time Magazine* January 21, 1991) is contradicted by two professors from Pennsylvania State's College of Medicine, who served on the Public Board of Inquiry on Depo Provera. As in Professor Toppozada's testimony, cited above, it is precisely their concern over the use of "progestogen alone as a contraceptive", whether in Depo Provera or Norplant, that prompted them to address "a major safety issue, that of carcinogenesis..." in a 1989 letter to the FDA commissioner.[7]

Norplant has been assumed to be safe because "Silicone rubber tubing has been used in surgical applications since the 1950s" (WHO 1990:3). However, this is problematic, particularly in light of current concerns over immune system disorders induced by breast implants. The health risks of silicone implantation, known to the manufacturers of the breast implants but hidden from consumers for almost two decades, were revealed after the adverse health effects of breast implants on women could no longer be ignored (*Washington Post* January 18, 1992). More generally, a team of researchers at the University of Texas have challenged the assumption that silicone elastomers used as medical implants and prostheses are generally inert. Based on testing of the same Silastic tubing used in Norplant, they describe their findings as "show[ing] that specific immune reactivity to elastomers of polydimethylsiloxane can develop in human beings" (Goldblum et al 1992:510). Even if Norplant promoters were to point to distinctions pertaining to the use of the Silastic casing in their implant, the burden of proof of long-term safety remains theirs. Indeed, to reiterate Katha Pollitt's call, "...let guinea pigs be the guinea pigs".

The variety of women's experiences with the New Reproductive Technology around the world, naturally, calls for different strategies for political activism appropriate to specific local agendas. Simultaneously, our concern with the social contexts of the use of this technology presents us with an opportunity for international cooperation. In this regard our pursuit of women's human rights, and the protection of our health requires more than individual attempts to demystify scientific knowledge or to bring international human rights law to bear on issues of reproductive rights (Coliver and Newman 1987). We must also consider variable cultural constructions of the "side effects" of pharmaceuticals (Etkin 1992) and hold individual physicians accountable for "betray[ing] medicine" (PHR 1992). We need nothing short of a collective, concerted effort in order to challenge the global power structures which produce misery among women "over here" and "over there". This requires informed solidarity as we struggle on behalf of ourselves, on our most accessible political turfs – in our own backyards – but also in egalitarian partnership with others around the globe. The victories of Bangladesh, Brazil, and California resonate in Egypt.

---

7 I acknowledge with gratitude the efforts of WEMOS in circulating copies of this letter.

References

Abdel Fadil M. "The Values of Progress, and the Values of Underdevelopment". *Al-Ahram Al-Iqtisadi* 1989; 1044 (January 16):20 (in Arabic).

ACLU. "ACLU Statement on Kansas HB 2089". *ACLU Reproductive Freedom Project* February, 1991.

ACLU. "Two More States Contemplate Punitive Welfare 'Reforms'". *Reproductive Rights Update* 1992; IV(7):6.

Alexander J. "Mobilizing against the state and international "aid" agencies: "third world" women define reproductive freedom". In *From Abortion to Reproductive Freedom: Transforming a Movement*. Ed. M. Gerber Fried. Boston: South End Press, 1990; 49-62.

Alvarez Martínez L. "A Latina Speaks on Choice". *The Network News* November/December 1992.

Amin, S. "Population and Development". *Socialist Review* 1976; 27:67-80.

Badran S. "Joint Research and the Myth of Transforming Egyptian Society". *Al-Tarbiyah al-Mu'asirah* 1984; 2:119-126 (in Arabic).

Baker B. "Sentenced to Norplant". *The Network News* January/February 1991.

BWHC [Boston Women's Health Book Collective]. *The New Our Bodies Ourselves*. New York: Simon and Schuster, 1984.

Coliver S. and Newman S. "Using International Human Rights Law to Influence United States Foreign Population Policy: Resort to Courts or Congress". *International Law and Politics* 1987; 20(53):53-91.

Cowley G. "A Birth-Control Breakthrough". *Newsweek* December 24, 1990.

Davis A. "Racism, birth control, and reproductive rights". In *From Abortion to Reproductive Freedom: Transforming a Movement*. Ed. M. Gerber Fried. Boston: South End Press 1990; 15-26.

Dickey C. "Egypt's Soaring Population Outstrips Efforts at Control". *Manchester Guardian Weekly*, January 12, 1986.

Dickson D. "Science and foreign policy: Knowledge as imperialism". In *The New Politics of Science*. New York: Pantheon Books 1984; 163-216.

Dobson T. "Medical Malpractice in the Birthplace: Resolving the Physician-Patient Conflict Through Informed Consent, Standard of Care, and Assumption of Risk". *Nebraska Law Review* 1986; (65):655-658.

Duster R. *Backdoor to Eugenics*. New York: Routledge, 1990.

El-Bayoumi A. "Answer to Dr Ibrahim Badran - Joint Research and the Scientific Method". *Al-Ahram Al-Iqtisadi* 1982; 22 (November 15).(In Arabic)

El-Bayoumi J. "Letter to the Editor". *Washington Post*, December 26, 1990.

El-Issawi I. *Population Explosion or Crisis of Development?* Cairo: Nationalist, Progressive Unionist Party, 1985 (in Arabic).

El-Sahwi M.S., Rizk M., Toppozada M. and Haiba N. "Experience with Norplant in Alexandria". In *Proceedings of the Symposium on Long-Term Subdermal Contraceptive Implants*. Ed. Shaaban M. Assiut: University of Assiut, 1984;10-19.

Escobar A. "Power and Visibility: Development and the Invention and Management of the Third World". *Cultural Anthropology* 1988; (3):428-443.

Etkin N. "'Side Effects': Cultural Constructions and Reinterpretations of Western Pharmaceuticals". *Medical Anthropology Quarterly* 1992; 6(2):99-113.

Ferris V.E. "Short Term Sterilization For the Reproductively Unfit". Unpublished paper prepared for Professor Kristin Luker's course on Law and Reproduction, University of California, Berkeley, 1991.

Galal D. *American Aid, For Who? Egypt or America?* Cairo: *Al-Ahram* Press, 1988 (in Arabic).

Gladwell, M. "Science Confronts Ethics In Contraceptive Implant". *The Washington Post*, October 31, 1990.

Goldblum R.M., Pelley R.P., O'Donell A.A., Pyron D., Heggers J.P. "Antibodies to Silicone Elastomers and Reactions to Ventriculoperitoneal Shunts". *Lancet* 1992; (340):510-513.

Haire D. *How the FDA Determines the 'Safety' of Drugs- Just How Safe is 'Safe'?* Washington, D.C.: NWHN, 1984.

Hammami R. and Rieker M. "Feminist Orientalism and Orientalist Marxism". *New Left Review* 1988; (170):93-109.

Hilts P.J. "Birth-Control Backlash". *The New York Times Magazine* December 16, 1990.

Hopkins N. *The Political Economy of an Upper Egyptian Village.* Unpublished manuscript draft, 1985.

Kennedy S. "Planning Tomorrow's Family". *Cairo Today*, 1986; (June): 24,31.

Ketchum S.A. Medicine and control of reproduction. In *Sexuality and Medicine: Ethical Viewpoints in Transition.* Ed. E.E Shelp. Dordrecht: Reidel Publishing Company 1987;17-38.

Kunstadter P. "Medical Ethics in Cross-Cultural and Multi-Cultural Perspectives". *Social Science and Medicine* 1980; (14B):289-296.

Lalevee T. "Egypt's Fight to Become the Japan of the Middle East". *Executive Intelligence Review*, December:30-32.

Leacock E. "Introduction". In *The Origin of the Family, Private Property and the State*. New York: International Publishers 1972.

Lewin T. "Implanted Birth Control Device Renews Debate Over Forced Contraception". *The New York Times*, January 10, 1991.

MacKenzie D. "Tackling Egypt's Baby Boom". *The Middle East* 1985; October, (132):51-52.

Mani L. "Multiple Mediations: Feminist Scholarship in the Age of Multinational Reception. *Feminist Review* 1990; (35):24-41.

Martin E. "The Cultural Construction of Gendered Bodies: Biology and Metaphors of Production and Destruction". Paper presented at the Annual Meeting of the American Anthropological Association, Phoenix, Arizona, Nov. 16-18, 1988.

Martinez E. "Caramba, Our Anglo Sisters Just Didn't Get It". *Network News* 1992, November/December 1,4-5.

Mohanty C.T. "Under Western Eyes: Feminist Scholarship and Colonial Discourse". *Boundary 2* 1984; 12(3)/(13(1): 33-358.

Mokhtar B. "Private Sector Family Planning". *An-Ahram* 1989; (January 3): 3.

Morsy S.A. *Social Dimensions of Norplant Use in Assiut: Report of a Preliminary Inquiry*. Unpublished report submitted to the Population Council and the Department of Obstetrics and Gynaecology, Assiut University: Faculty of Medicine, June 1985.

Morsy S.A. "U.S. Aid to Egypt: An Illustration and Account of U.S. Foreign Assistance Policy". *Arab Studies Quarterly* 1986a; 8(4):358-389.

Morsy S.A. "Implant Contraception and Family Planning: Between Propaganda and Serious Evaluation". *Al-Mar'a Al-Gadida* 1986b; July.

Morsy S.A. "Implant Contraception as a Human Rights Issue". Panel Discussion on *Pharmaceuticals and Human Rights.* Alexandria Association of Human Rights Advocates, October 1986c.

Morsy S.A. "Safeguarding Women's Bodies : The White Man's Burden Medicalized". *Medical Anthropology Quarterly* 1991; 5(1):19-23.

Murray W. "Assembly Bill No. 3559". *California Legislature - 1991-92 Regular Session*. February 21, 1992.

Noble Tesh S. *Hidden Arguments*. Rutgers: Rutgers University Press, 1989.

NWHN "The Cervical Cap- Here at Last". *The Network Newsletter* 1988; (May/June): 1-3.

NWHN (National Women's Health Network). "Testimony Before the Fertility and Maternal Health Drugs Advisory Committee of the Food and Drug Administration by Judy Norsigian, National Women Health Network, April 27, 1989". *Network News*, November/December,

PHR (Physicians for Human Rights) "When Doctors Betray Medicine". *Record* 1992; V(2):8.

Pollitt K. "Implants: Truth and Consequences". *The Nation* 1992; 254(10):325,329.

Population Information Program (The Johns Hopkins University). "Hormonal contraception: New Long-Lasting Methods". *Population Reports* 1987; Series K(3):58.

Kaplan G. "An Afternoon with Anwar el-Sadat". *Institutional Investor*. August 1976.

Price L. "A Medical Anthropologist's Ruminations on NIH Funding". *Medical Anthropology Quarterly* 1992; (692):128-146.

Purvis A. "A Pill That Gets Under the Skin". *Time* December 24, 1990.

Rakusen J. "Depo-Provera, the extent of the problem: Case study in the politics of birth control". In *Women, Health and Reproduction*. Eds. Robert H., Routledge and Kegan Paul, 1981: 88.

Reis A. *Contraception: Professionals Take Away Women's Control*. Unpublished manuscript, n.d.

Rose S. "Scientific racism and ideology: the IQ racket from Galton to Jensen". In *The Political Economy of Science: Ideology of/in the Natural Sciences*. Eds. Rose H. and Rose S. London: MacMillan Press, 1976.

Rose H. and Hamner J. "Women's liberation: reproduction and the technological fix". In *The Political Economy of Science: Ideology of/in the Natural Sciences*. Eds. Rose H. and Rose S. London: MacMillan Press, London, 1976.

Said A.M. et al. "Experience With Norplant in Zagazig". In *Proceedings of the Symposium on Long-Term Subdermal Contraceptive Implants.* Ed. Shaaban M. Assiut: University of Assiut, 1984: 28-39.

Salah M. *Acceptability of Contraception by Norplant Among Egyptian Women.* [Doctoral Thesis] Assiut: Assiut University, Faculty of Medicine, Department of Obstetrics and Gynecology, 1983.

Salem H.T., Abdulla K.A. and Shaaban M.M. "Norplant and Lactation". In *Proceedings of the Symposium on Long-Term Subdermal Contraceptive Implants.* Ed. Shaaban M. Assiut: University of Assiut, 1984:139-150.

Shaaban M. and Salah M. "A Two-Year Experience with Norplant in Assiut". In *Proceedings of the Symposium on Long-Term Subdermal Contraceptive Implants.* Ed. Shaaban M. Assiut: University of Assiut, 1984:23-24.

Shaaban M. ed. *Proceedings of the Symposium on Long-Term Subdermal Contraceptive Implants.* Ed. Shaaban M. Assiut: University of Assiut, 1984.

Shapiro T. *Population Control Politics: Women, Sterilization, and Reproductive Choice.* Philadelphia: Temple University Press, 1985.

Sholkamy H.M. *They Are the Government: Bureaucracy in an Egyptian Village.* [MA Thesis] American University in Cairo, Department of Sociology-Anthropology, 1988:149.

UBINIG *Norplant: The Five Year Needle.* Policy Research for Development Alternatives, Bangladesh, 1988.

White E.C., ed. *The Black Woman's Health Book: Speaking for Ourselves.* The Seal Press, 1990.

WHO. "Facts About an Implantable Contraceptive: Memorandum from a WHO Meeting". *Bulletin of the World Health Organization* (63):485-494.

WHO *Norplant Contraceptive Subdermal Implants: Managerial and Technical Guidelines* (Provisional Version). Geneva, 1990.

Yanoshik K. and Norsigian J. "Contraception, control, and choice: International perspectives". In *Healing Technology: Feminist Perspectives.* Ed. Strother Ratcliff K. Ann Arbor: University of Michigan Press, 1989.

Conclusion

From the standpoint of women's control over their lives, Norplant's design is unsettling. Six capsules are implanted into a woman's arm and release a hormone which prevents pregnancy until she has the capsules surgically removed. Women do not need to remember to do anything to avoid pregnancy, like taking a pill daily or using a barrier method during sex. However, women also cannot start or stop using the method on their own. The design of Norplant ultimately takes these decisions and puts them into the hands of the health worker who must surgically insert or remove the method. The woman who uses Norplant must ask for removal. Ideally, she should never be refused or pressured into changing her mind. Even under ideal conditions, however, she is dependent upon someone else if she chooses to stop using this contraceptive.

The articles in this book describe how Norplant has been administered and used in different settings. It is apparent from these reports that women's reproductive rights are not always upheld. In Indonesia, high prices were used to dissuade women from having Norplant removed prior to five years; in Brazil, women were not followed up and could not find a doctor trained to remove Norplant five to six years after it was inserted; and in Thailand, women were not informed that they had contradictions to Norplant use and had it inserted in spite of these contraindications.

The article from Finland presents a setting in which health care providers try to give women a free and informed choice by providing counselling on the effects and potential side-effects of the method. Most of the health care providers and medical experts interviewed regard Norplant as a second choice contraceptive technology to be used if other methods such as the contraceptive pill or the IUD are not suitable. The respondents recommended it as an appropriate method for "asocial" women who forget to use the pill regularly or are alcoholics or psychiatric patients. In the US, Norplant has been proposed for welfare mothers and a woman convicted of child abuse. These reports raise concerns of double standards. Is Norplant to be a first choice method for women in developing countries and women who face discrimination in industrialised countries, but a second choice method for other women in industrialised countries?

The lack of recognition of women's reproductive rights described in most of the contributions to this book is unacceptable. Why this discrepancy between the principle of free and informed choice, and practice? One explanation is the primary goal of many family planning programmes to reduce population growth, not to genuinely meet women's needs. Another reason is the professional attitude of health care providers in many settings: they are the experts and believe that they know what is best for women. In "persuading" women to use Norplant they feel that they are doing good. Social attitudes towards women also make it easier to dismiss some of the "normal" side-effects of Norplant – menstrual cycle disturbances, headaches, and psychological effects – as unimportant, even in cultural settings in which they have a large effect on women's social and community life.

Medicalisation of side-effects

The WHO and Population Council manuals on Norplant advise against medical treatment of the menstrual disturbances resulting from Norplant use. However, in both the Finnish and Indonesian study health care providers treated these disturbances with medicines. In Finland physicians prescribed progestins and/or oestrogens and in the Indonesian study health workers prescribed Vitamin K and the physician prescribed oestrogens. These are ad hoc treatments using pharmaceuticals for purposes for which they have never been tested and which are not on their official lists of indications. The effects of combined hormonal therapies (higher doses of progestins or combined oestrogen/progestin pills and progestin implants) on a woman's health are unknown, particularly if she receives combined treatments during the early weeks or months of Norplant use, when the daily release of levonorgestrel is highest. This is also a further medicalisation of healthy women following Norplant use. Women are given one synthetic hormone as a contraceptive; they are then treated with another hormone or vitamin because of the side-effects of the first. A simpler solution would be to remove the cause of the problem.

Furthermore, in Finland most providers first prescribe mini-pills to test their client's reaction to progestin-only contraception – a practice which is not appropriate because the predictive value of the mini-pill for side-effects from Norplant has not yet been assessed.

Lack of access to removal

The reports from Indonesia, Thailand and Brazil indicate that it is generally easier to have Norplant inserted than to have it removed. In Lombok health staff tried to convince women to continue to use the method because of the financial loss to the family planning programme if the full five years of efficacy are not completed. In Brazil, 14 out of 52 women interviewed still had Norplant implanted more than five years after insertion, past the time when it should have been removed. They had not been contacted for removal and there were no trained staff in the local health centre who could remove the implants after the discontinuation of the Norplant trial.

In Egypt, six instances were reported of women taking part in an introductory trial who were refused removal of Norplant. The report illustrates how the response of women to this refusal can differ. One woman went to on "outside" doctor in search of removal, while another woman accepted the situation and tried to endure the side-effects of the contraceptive.

In Finland, women have free access to removal facilities; however most of the physicians interviewed reported that they had experienced difficulties in removing the implants because of incorrect insertion or breaking of rods during removal.

The lack of access to removal facilities and the problems encountered in the removal process itself indicate the importance of considering the provider-dependent and complex nature of Norplant when deciding whether to introduce the technology into a new health care setting. Another important consideration is whether health care services can follow up women for five years to ensure that they have Norplant removed or replaced when it is no longer effective.

Norplant and the user

All of the authors mention concerns about the effects of the menstrual disturbances caused by Norplant on the general well-being of women.

In Lombok, Hanhart reports that women worry about amenorrhoea (the absence of bleeding), fearing that they will become ill due to the unclean blood staying in their bodies. They are also affected by too abundant or too frequent bleeding because this requires them to wash themselves more often and because during bleeding they cannot have intercourse with their husbands. Even though the women in Lombok are reassured by the health workers, who state that the change in menstrual patterns is "normal",

Hanhart suggests that Norplant often affects women's general well-being adversely. She comments that women do not easily talk about menstruation and sexuality with health workers, and for this reason will not always report their feelings about the changes in their bleeding patterns. The structured surveys that are usually done to assess Norplant's acceptability are therefore not likely to result in accurate assessments of women's satisfaction.

The report from Brazil also mentions the women's dislike of the irregular menstrual bleeding pattern because they generally feel that it is bad to have sex when one is menstruating.

Some women in Brazil also reported lowered libido due to Norplant use. In both Egypt and Brazil, women mention mood changes and depression from Norplant use. The Egyptian report stresses the difference in the way scientists and health workers interpret side-effects as compared to users. The menstrual disturbances are considered normal by the providers of contraceptive method, while users are frequently seriously bothered by these adverse effects. The researchers from Brazil comment that Norplant changes the concept of what a "normal" menstrual pattern is. When women are worried about changes in menstruation caused by Norplant, health workers assure them that these are "normal".

Both the Finnish and the Egyptian report mention the role of the popular press in promoting the new technology. Women in both countries appear to be attracted to use Norplant by misleadingly positive media reports. The reality of Norplant use can then be rather a disappointment.

Conclusion

In future evaluations of Norplant's appropriateness, researchers should address the following priority issues apart from the usual monitoring of health indicators and acceptability:

1. *The recognition of women's reproductive rights in the provision of Norplant*:
   - Are women given a free and informed choice out of a range of contraceptives?
   - Do health care providers promote the method as a first choice method, safer and more effective than existing methods, or do they adequately inform women about advantages and disadvantages of each of the methods?
   - Are the same medical standards for safe use applied in developing countries as in industrialised countries?

- Is there a difference in standards applied to minority or disadvantaged women within an industrialised or developing country?

2. *The effect of menstrual disturbances on women's lives, sexual practices and libido:*
   - Is Norplant adversely affecting the quality of women's daily lives?
   - Do women find menstrual cycle disturbances acceptable?
   - How frequently do women experience decreased libido?

3. *Medicalisation of side-effects:*
   - Do health care providers treat the side-effects of Norplant with hormones and other medicines? Have the safety and effectiveness of these treatments been tested?

4. *Sterile technique:*
   - Is proper sterile technique used at all times to ensure that blood and/or contaminated instruments do not expose women to HIV or Hepatitis B infections during insertions or removals?

5. *Access to removal services:*
   - Can a health service ensure that women have free access to removal of Norplant when they request it and that no financial or other barriers prevent this?
   - What problems occur during the removal process?

6. *Adequate long-term follow-up:*
   - Can a health service adequately follow up women for five years to ensure that women have Norplant capsules removed or replaced when they are no longer effective?

7. *The promotion of Norplant in women's magazines and in the national press:*
   - What is written about Norplant in the popular media?
   - How adequate is the information provided?
   - Is it biased and promotional?

The Population Council, the US-based non-governmental organisation which developed Norplant and provides technical assistance for its introduction, recognizes the need for care in introducing Norplant because of its design.

Karen Beattie states that the Population Council seeks settings for the introduction of Norplant where women can receive: (Beattie 1992)

- a real choice of methods;
- accurate, balanced information;
- an easy relationship with the service provider;
- gentle correct insertion;
- sensitive management of problems;
- access to removal on demand;
- five year removal.

According to Beattie, the Population Council cannot ensure that Norplant is only provided in these types of settings. They advise countries on Norplant introduction; the actual implementation of family planning programmes remains under the sovereignty of national governments (Beattie 1992, pers comm).

As developers and advisors, however, the Population Council could take a more active role to ensure that these guidelines are met. For example, they could withdraw financial support for introductory programmes which do not meet these conditions, especially where serious problems continue to occur in spite of efforts to improve the situation; they could recommend against licensing and registration of Norplant in countries which have not met these guidelines during introductory trials; they could more actively monitor both trials and family planning programmes providing Norplant for infringements of human rights and, where infringements are found to occur, they could make their findings public and pressure publicly for change.

How frequently are these conditions met?

The case studies from developing countries in this book do not give a complete overview of the situation in each country. However, they present a disturbing indication of instances in which these conditions set by the Population Council are not being met. This has occured during introductory trials (Brazil and Egypt), training (Thailand) and provision within a family planning programme (Indonesia). This has also been documented elsewhere, as reported in some of the acceptability studies of Norplant (Zimmerman et al. 1990).

What can be done about this discrepancy between theory and practice?

The first priority is to upgrade the quality of contraceptive services. Family planning programmes need to be reoriented towards meeting the fertility needs of women and men and being responsive to the effect of contraceptives on the general well-being of users. The success of a family planning service should be measured in terms of quality of services and user satisfaction, not in numbers of contraceptives provided.

Such upgrading of services requires resources and time. In many developing countries budgets for health services are diminishing instead of increasing, reflecting a worsening economic situation and the need to repay debts. Additionally, health and social services have been cut within structural adjustment programmes imposed by the World Bank and International Monetary Fund as a precondition for loans.

In many countries, rapid improvement of the quality of health care services is unlikely. Therefore, the contraceptive technologies available need to be adjusted to fit existing services. If the quality of services or respect for reproductive rights within services is poor, methods which are administered by health workers or which require extensive follow-up care for proper use should be avoided. One can question the selection of complex, provider dependent contraceptive methods for widespread distribution in such countries. The cost of a method like Norplant also needs to be considered, particularly if it leads family planning workers to inform women that, because of the cost, they must keep Norplant in for the full five years of efficacy. This has occurred in Thailand and in Indonesia (Zimmerman et al. 1990; Hanhart, this book).

Why have family planning administrators not promoted simpler, user-controlled technologies such as the condom and the diaphragm, backed up by safe abortion services in case of method failure? An evaluation of the appropriateness of all existing contraceptive technologies is needed in relation to the quality of existing health care and family planning services, and the effects of each method on the general well-being of women and men within the context of the society in which they live. The advantages and disadvantages of new technologies such as Norplant should be compared to other contraceptives already on the market, including user-controlled contraceptives.

Planning for contraceptive development and implementation of family planning programmes must be changed to incorporate the views of the women – and hopefully men – who are using or will eventually use contraceptives. This requires a major reorientation of the goals of contraceptive development towards the needs of users. It is not enough to carry out research on reproductive physiology and develop a method which can prevent pregnancy as effectively as possible with few serious health risks. Acceptability studies which look mainly at rates of continued use are also not enough. Users must be involved from the start in defining what kinds of methods they need. Acceptability needs to be defined much more broadly to include effects on well-being and on human rights.

Norplant was developed to have certain qualities: high effectiveness over a long period of time. These are useful qualities for family planning services which aim to reduce population growth quickly. However, the trade-off has been lack of control by women and a high frequency of side-effects affecting daily life.

Policy makers from countries which have not yet introduced Norplant need to consider whether it provides an advantage over existing contraceptives. Can they meet the Population Council's guidelines for service delivery, including removal on request? Can they afford the cost of providing Norplant in the long run, including the cost of follow-up of users and continued training in insertion and removal?

If Norplant cannot be provided safely and respectfully and with a woman's fully informed consent, it should not be provided. It is not enough to say that certain conditions must be met, but to turn a blind eye when they are not met; Norplant has a design which makes it prone to abuse because of the need for surgery for removal. Policy makers, donor agencies and non-governmental organisations (NGOs) involved in contraceptive development have a role to play in ensuring that the needs and well-being of contraceptive users come first.

References

Beattie K. "Introduction of New Contraceptive Method: An Opportunity for Promoting the User's Perspective in Family Planning Programmes." *A Question of Control.* ed. Barbara Mintzes. WEMOS/HAI, 1992.

Population Council. Personal communation. K. Beattie. October 30, 1992.

Zimmerman M., Haffey J., Crane E., et al. "Assessing the Acceptability of Norplant Implants in Four Countries: Findings from Focus Group Discussions." *Studies in Family Planning*, 1990; 21(2): 21-103.

Notes on the authors

Solange Gandur Dacach is a sociologist and feminist. She is one of the founders of Rede de Defesa da Especie Humana (REDEH), where she works as educational coordinator. She has been active for 15 years in the field of Reproductive Rights doing research and working with action groups.

Giselle Raquel Garcia is a physician specialised in psychiatry and public health. She is a feminist and co-founder of REDEH, where she is the research coordinator. She has been active in the field of women's health and rights for 12 years, in independent groups as well as in the public sector.

Jannemieke Hanhart has a degree in social work and worked with mentally and physically handicapped people for four years in public health in Amsterdam. The field study on Norplant in Indonesia was conducted as part of her MA thesis (Social Anthropology, University of Amsterdam). She is currently interim coordinator for the Women's Health Action Foundation (WHAF).

Anita Hardon is a medical biologist in the Medical Anthropology Unit of the University of Amsterdam. She conducted research on the use and distribution of pharmaceuticals in the Philippines between 1985 and 1988. Her present research interests include pharmaceutical cost-recovery, contraceptives and injections. She was a co-founder of the Women & Pharmaceuticals Project and is currently working as research coordinator.

Elina Hemminki is a physician and senior researcher for the Academy of Finland. Current research interests include evaluation of health services for women, especially reproductive technologies.

Kristiina Kajesalo is a physician, currently working in a centre for alcoholics and drug addicts. Her interests are women, health and the Third World.

Prasert Kiatboonsri is a pharmacist who worked for a number of years as a public health researcher with the Drug Information for Action Centre in Bangkok. He was co-editor of the centre's bulletin, which aimed to portray the role of medicine from a socio-political perspective.

Barbara Mintzes worked for seven years as a community health educator at the Vancouver Women's Health Collective, a Canadian feminist women's health centre. She has been active in DES Action Canada since 1983 and currently works at the European office of Health Action International in Amsterdam.

Soheir Morsy is a medical anthropologist. Following undergraduate training in Bacteriology, she held technical positions at the Department of Biological Sciences and the Institute of Molecular Biophysics of Florida State University, and later at the Department of Biophysics of MIT. In Egypt she taught Science at El-Nasr Girls' College in Alexandria. After graduate training in Medical Anthropology she taught at Michigan State University, the American University in Cairo, and most recently, the University of California, Berkeley.

Eeva Ollila is a physician, currently working as a researcher in the Department of Public Health at the University of Helsinki. The main topic of her research is Norplant. She is an activist in the Third World Movement, Physicians for Social Responsibility and Health Action International.

Piengporn Panut-Ampon is a micro-biologist by training. She was the coordinator of an integrated health project in Thai villages and co-editor of the Drug Information for Action Centre Bulletin for Thai health professionals.

Judith Richter is a pharmacist and health activist who is currently working as a freelance researcher. She worked for four and a half years in Thailand as a lecturer in Community Pharmacy and a team member of a Thai public interest group (Drug Information for Action Centre). Her main interests are the international politics of pharmaceuticals, women and reproductive technologies, communication and power.

Publications

Women's Health Action Foundation and WEMOS

Marketing Fertility
Ivan Wolffers, Anita Hardon and Janita Janssen (eds.)
A critical examination of the promotion and use of high dose oestrogen progestin drugs. Available in Dutch and English.
1989 WEMOS, Women and Pharmaceuticals Project (dfl. 17.50)

RU 486: The Abortion Pill
Proceedings of a seminar on the abortion pill, Amsterdam 1990.
1990 WEMOS, Women and Pharmaceuticals Project (dfl. 15.00)

Women and Pharmaceuticals Bulletin
Women and Pharmaccuticals Group (eds.)
Contains articles on reproductive technologies including DES, Norplant, the contraceptive vaccine and the abortion pill, as well as a critical review of clinical trials of contraceptives.
1990 WEMOS, Women and Pharmaceuticals Project and HAI (dfl.10.00)

Guidelines for the distribution and use of fertility regulating technologies.
These guidelines have been formulated in consultation with and on request of women and health groups in developing countries. They contain criteria for the safe and ethical provision of fertility regulating methods centred on the needs of users. In English and Spanish.
1991 WEMOS, Women and Pharmaceuticals Project (dfl. 5.00)

A Question of Control. Women's perspectives on the development and use of contraceptives.
Barbara Mintzes (ed.)
Report of an international conference, April 1991. It contains a selection of presentations and discussions on contraceptive research and the use and provision of contraceptives, viewed from a perspective which centres on the needs and desires of the user, rather than the desire to control population growth.
1992 WEMOS, Women and Pharmaceuticals Project and HAI (dfl.20.00)

Exposed: Deadly Export. The story of European Community exports of banned or withdrawn drugs to the Third World.
Bas van der Heide
This publication gives the results of a survey of drugs banned or withdrawn in one or more EC-countries which were for sale in Africa, the Caribbean, the Middle East or Asia in 1988. The WEMOS Pharma Project calls for a stricter export legislation at a national and European level.
1991 WEMOS, Pharma Project. (dfl. 10.00 for individuals and non-profit institutions and dfl. 50.00 for others)

Shipping and handling costs not included. Publications are available at reduced rates to groups in developing countries. For more information or details, please write to:

WOMEN'S HEALTH ACTION FOUNDATION
P.O. Box 4263
1009 AG Amsterdam
The Netherlands